Neuroplasticity

The Secret Behind Brain Plasticity

(A Cognitive Behavioral Approach to Anxiety and Procrastination)

Johnnie Cantrell

Published By **Elena Holly**

Johnnie Cantrell

*Neuroplasticity: The Secret Behind Brain Plasticity
(A Cognitive Behavioral Approach to Anxiety and
Procrastination)*

ISBN 978-1-7774626-1-1

No part of this guidebook shall be reproduced in any form without permission in writing from the publisher except in the case of brief quotations embodied in critical articles or reviews.

Legal & Disclaimer

Table Of Contents

Chapter 1: Understanding The Human Brain

From the historical Egyptians who pioneered the technique of mummification to the medical discoveries of the 18th century getting to know "globules" and neurons, neurology has an extended and illustrious data. Sadly, inside the early days of civilization, effective units for analyzing the human thoughts were restricted, and assumptions about its inner workings had been often wrong. The mind changed into once notion to be cranial fluff. The coronary heart, in preference to the mind, emerge as seemed because of the reality the wellspring of thoughts in ancient Egypt, fundamental to its elimination at some stage in mummification preparations starting inside the overdue Middle Kingdom.

According to Herodotus, the famous Greek historian, the primary diploma of mummification modified into casting off the thoughts as very well as feasible with an iron hook, with any residual materials blended with drug treatments. During the following 5 millennia, this factor of view superior, and the thoughts came to be noted because of the fact the net website of thoughts, but remnants of the old idea that the coronary heart grow to be the center of human intelligence persist in idiomatic phrases inclusive of "memorizing some thing by way of coronary heart."

Let us start with the historical Egyptians and feature a observe some of the most massive advances in our information of the human thoughts at some point of records.

Beyond the Skull in Egypt

The Edwin Smith Surgical Papyrus, which dates lower back to the 17th century BC, has the oldest recorded connection with the mind. The hieroglyph for the brain occurs eight times in this papyrus, outlining the signs and signs, evaluation, and analysis of patients with head wounds and complex fractures of the cranium. According to the author's judgments as a fight doctor, historic Egyptians had a hazy draw near of the consequences of mind trauma. While the signs and symptoms are exact in complete, there can be no medical priority. The author notices "the pulsations of the exposed mind" and compares the thoughts's floor to the undulating floor of copper slag, which does, in truth, show a gyral-sulcal sample.

The Edwin Smith Surgical Papyrus has big documentation on the relationship most of the element of damage and the accompanying signs, which incorporates aphasia ("he talks now not to thee") and seizures ("he shudders excessively") after head trauma. These records, at the same time as indicating a essential hobby of the underlying mechanics and the want of protective the cranium, handiest provide a less than extremely good photo of the human brain's complexity. Given that previous civilizations' scientific strategies were primarily based completely mostly on myths and superstitions, the battlefield health practitioner's observations appear like empirical and based completely totally on logical reasoning and simple commentary.

When the ancient Egyptians observed the human thoughts for the number one time at the same time as the man or woman changed into even though alive, they did no longer regard it due to the truth the center of mind and emotion. Indeed, as previously said, at the same time as making prepared a person for mummification, they would collapse the thoughts thru pushing a metal straw into the throat.

The Ancient Greeks Argue Over the Function of the Brain

The Ancient Greeks had a hobby with the mind, which commenced out with Alcmaeon's pioneering study. In his studies, Alcmaeon dissected the eye and proposed a link among the mind and vision. He additionally stated that the thoughts, now not the coronary coronary heart, had dominion over the body (a notion ultimately renamed the hegemonikon by using the usage of Stoics) and that the senses had been dependent on the thoughts. According to Alcmaeon, the functionality of the thoughts to synthesize senses is the foundation of its function as the center of memory and mind. Similarly, the writer of On the Holy Illness, a component of the Hippocratic corpus, advocated the brain because the seat of mind.

The debate over the hegemonikon raged on for a long time among historical Greek philosophers and scientific docs. Aristotle proposed in the fourth century BC that the coronary coronary coronary heart became the middle of thoughts and the mind was exceptional a cooler for the blood. He reasoned that people have been more logical than animals because of the fact they'd huge brains to mild their warm-bloodedness, amongst different factors. In assessment, Herophilus and Erasistratus of Alexandria went on a journey including the dissection of human our our bodies in the course of the Hellenistic technology, providing proof of the mind's prominent significance. Their research led them to distinguish the cerebrum from the cerebellum, further to to perceive the ventricles and the dura mater. While their writings have normally been out of place to the annals of time, their achievements had been exceeded down thru secondary property. Some of their findings had been not rediscovered till millennia after they died.

Galen-Dissection of the Brain

During the Roman Empire's heyday, the great Greek medical doctor and fact seeker Galen investigated the mysteries of the mind via the usage of dissecting the brains of non-human animals including oxen, Barbary apes, and pigs. Galen deduced from his findings that the cerebellum, which come to be thicker than the thoughts, commanded the muscle tissues, while the cerebrum, which changed into softer, have become in rate of decoding sensory statistics. He moreover advocated that the thoughts labored with the beneficial aid of the drift of animal spirts thru the

6

ventricles. Galen also identified that certain spinal nerves dominated particular muscle businesses and theorized muscular reciprocity. Only in the nineteenth century, with the groundbreaking artwork of François Magendie and Charles Bell, did the facts of spinal function surpass Galen's.

As we hold our journey through time, leaving the Roman Empire and into Medieval durations, we notice that our statistics of the mind is progressively developing. But, it changed into now not till the Middle Ages that subjects commenced out to take shape in the realm of neurology.

Islamic Medicine within the Middle Ages and Mental Health

Islamic treatment become focused in the Middle Ages with clarifying the complex courting among the thoughts and frame and spotting the want of expertise highbrow nicely-being. Al-Zahrawi, who lived in Islamic Iberia in the one year a thousand, assessed patients with neurological issues and achieved surgical techniques for head traumas, cranium fractures, spinal injuries, hydrocephalus, subdural effusions, and headaches.

Avicenna, additionally known as Ibn-Sina in Persia, modified right right into a excellent student who changed into well-versed in skull fractures and related surgical remedies. Some regard him to be the father of modern-day remedy. He wrote 40 treatises on medication, the most well-known of which come to be the Qanun, a systematic compendium that became utilized in universities for over a century. Insomnia, mania, hallucinations, nightmares, dementia, epilepsy, stroke, paralysis, vertigo, melancholia, and tremors were all covered in his books. Avicenna additionally located Junun Mufrit, a sickness similar to schizophrenia. Agitation, sleep problems, wrong replies to queries, and intermittent loss of speech have been all signs and symptoms of the disorder. Avicenna moreover diagnosed the cerebellar vermis, which he actually known as the vermis, and the caudate nucleus. Both phrases are although applied in neuroanatomy in recent times. He have become additionally the number one to hyperlink highbrow troubles to faults inside the mind's center ventricle or frontal lobe.

Abulcasis, Averroes, Avenzoar, and Maimonides all studied mind-associated scientific worries inside the direction of the Medieval Muslim international. Meanwhile, European scientists started out their private studies into human anatomy, which covered painstakingly documenting the human mind. Mondino de Luzzi and Guido da Vigevano wrote the primary anatomy textbooks in Europe, which protected an entire explanation of the brain, most of the 13th and 14th centuries.

The Scientific Revolution And The Renaissance

Andreas Vesalius exposed issues with the conventional Galenic attitude on anatomy at some point of his examinations of human cadavers. Vesalius thoroughly documented numerous anatomical features of each the thoughts and the general annoying system at some point of his dissections. Along with describing a slew of bodily systems similar to the putamen and corpus callosum, Vesalius proposed that the brain modified into made up of seven pairs of 'mind nerves,' every having its private motive. Subsequent researchers contributed their very very personal complex depictions of the human mind to Vesalius' pioneering artwork.

In the 17th century, René Descartes dedicated himself to reading the body shape of the mind, providing the dualism speculation to deal with the question of ways the thoughts hyperlinks to the thoughts. After coming across the thoughts's strategies answerable for the flow into of cerebrospinal fluid, Descartes claimed that the pineal gland functioned because the vicinity wherein the thoughts interacted with the frame. Jan Swammerdam did an check in the course of the identical time in which he inserted frog thigh muscle in an hermetic syringe with a touch quantity of water inside the tip. By stimulating the nerve to reason muscular contraction, he located that the water degree did no longer upward push as expected, therefore disproving the balloonist notion.

The idea that nerve stimulation induced movement has large implications because it proposed that conduct is grounded in inputs. Thomas Willis studied the mind, nerves, and conduct inside the mid-1600s in an try and increase remedies for neurological ailments. His take a look at covered a detailed description of the anatomy of the brainstem, cerebellum, ventricles, and cerebral hemispheres.

Electricity and Neurons inside the 1700s and 1800s

Luigi Galvani, Lucia Galeazzi Galvani, and Giovanni Aldini have been the number one to find out the presence of power in nerves ultimately of their dissection of frogs within the 2nd a part of the 18th century. Yet, as we are able to see on this segment, it became not till the nineteenth century that our understanding of the thoughts expert a dramatic shift.

César Julien Jean Legallois completed the floor-breaking achievement of delineating the particular cause of a brain region in 1811. He studied breathing the use of animal dissection and lesions and determined the middle of breathing in the medulla oblongata. Meanwhile, between 1811 and 1824, Charles Bell and François Magendie completed dissections and vivisections that determined out motor impulse transmission via the ventral roots of the spine and sensory input reception through the posterior roots (Bell-Magendie law).

Jean Pierre Flourens pioneered the use of focused lesions of the mind in animals and located the effects on motility, sensitivity, and conduct within the 1820s. He determined that eliminating the cerebellum led to disorganized and erratic motions. Later, inside the mid-1800s, Emil du Bois-Reymond,

Johannes Peter Müller, and Hermann von Helmholtz located that neurons had been electrically excitable and that their hobby ought to constantly effect the electrical country of neighboring neurons.

In their try and recognize the mind, researchers frequently flip to people who've had severe thoughts harm. Phineas Gage, for example, have turn out to be impaled by way of the usage of an iron rod in his frontal lobe at some point of a blasting accident in 1848. Gage's instance changed into described with the aid of John Martyn Harlow, who located key hyperlinks most of the prefrontal thoughts and executive capabilities. Similarly, Paul Broca noticed a affected person in 1861 who had out of place speech and paralysis but preserved facts and intellectual capacity. Broca did an autopsy and positioned a lesion inside the affected individual's frontal lobe inside the left cerebral hemisphere, which brought about his seminal ebook at the challenge. Others had been endorsed with the aid of the use of Broca's artwork to conduct

13

meticulous post-mortem so as to narrate new thoughts regions to sensory and motor strategies.

The localization concept of mind function have become in big element diagnosed in the late nineteenth century. Gustav Fritsch and Eduard Hitzig showed that activating certain sections of a canine's motor cortex induced involuntary muscle contractions in numerous quantities of the body, constructing at the art work of Broca and others. In the 1870s, John Hughlings Jackson as it must be decided the structure of the motor cortex with the useful resource of tracking the path of seizures in epileptic patients. Carl Wernicke extended on Broca's findings, presenting a mind location specialized for language comprehension and creation. Richard Caton investigated the electric interest of the cerebral hemispheres in rabbits and monkeys in 1875. Hermann Munk, David Ferrier, and Harvey Cushing all contributed considerably to our knowledge of vision, audition, and touch localization in the occipital, advanced temporal, and postcentral gyrus, respectively.

Advances in microscopy and staining strategies enabled a more unique exam of the thoughts within the late 19th century. The neuron doctrine changed into developed because of Camillo Golgi's use of silver chromate salt staining, which indicates that the neuron is the sensible unit of the brain. In 1906, Santiago Ramón y Cajal and Golgi shared the Nobel Prize in Physiology or Medicine for his or her discoveries at the shape and characteristic of neurons. Galvani's have a examine on the electric excitability of muscle tissues and neurons moreover helped to make clean the neuron idea. Moreover, in 1898, John Newport Langley used the word "autonomic" to explain the connections of nerve fibers to peripheral nerve cells. He is also stated for his contributions to chemical receptor concept and the belief of "receptive substance."

By the end of the nineteenth century, the clinical global had completed an intensive keep near of the inner workings of the neurological machine, due in massive difficulty to the pioneering paintings of Francis Gotch. Gotch stated a vital phenomena referred to as the "inexcitable" or "refractory period" that takes place amongst nerve impulses in 1899. His investigations in large element targeted at the impact of nerve interconnections on muscle and ocular characteristic, losing glowing slight on the relationship the numerous involved machine and the body.

Yet this have become surely the begin of a adventure that would lead us well past a rudimentary keep near of the shape and function of the thoughts. With the arrival of the 20 th century came an explosion of scientific manipulation strategies, permitting us to dive deeper than ever before into the secrets of the thoughts. Modern neuroscience has transformed our know-how of the brain and the way we approach mind-related medical problems, from early electroencephalography (EEG) machines that allowed us to hit upon and look at mind hobby to the most superior neuroimaging strategies that permit us to visualize the mind's internal workings in splendid element.

We want to count on many greater advances within the destiny years as we artwork to locate the secrets and strategies of the thoughts and harness its capability to decorate our health and nicely-being.

From the Twentieth Century to the Present

Neuroscience arose as an precise and cohesive educational discipline in the 20th century, brilliant from exceptional medical areas. Previous to this, the take a look at of the worried device emerge as often seen as a subset of various fields of studies. This new forte allowed for a more emphasis at the hectic device and its intricacies, resulting in massive advancements within the region. Researchers have been able to dive deeper into the complexity of the mind way to this multiplied emphasis on neuroscience, generating new strategies and technology to better our expertise.

Ivan Pavlov made an indelible mark on neurophysiology. His studies were especially concerned with temperament, training, and reflex responses. In 1891, Pavlov have end up invited to the Institute of Experimental Medicine in St. Petersburg, wherein he emerge as in rate of organising and handling the Department of Physiology. Pavlov released The Work of the Digestive Glands in 1897, after 12 years of significant trying out, incomes him the renowned Nobel Prize in Physiology and Medicine in 1904. Pavlov's discoveries no longer extremely good stronger our information of the digestive device, however additionally of the neurological tool and its link to behavior.

Vladimir Bekhterev made giant contributions to neurophysiology in the early twentieth century through figuring out 15 new reflexes and competing with Pavlov within the research of conditioned reflexes. In 1907, Bekhterev mounted the Psychoneurological Institute in St. Petersburg, wherein he cooperated with Alexandre Dogiel to increase a multidisciplinary technique to analyzing the brain. On July 14, 1950, extra than 4 many years later, the Institute of Higher Nervous Activity became based in Moscow, Russia, furthering our data of the neurological machine.

Charles Scott Sherrington made vast contributions to the take a look at of reflexes and motor gadgets in the early 20th century. He used the time period synapses to describe the unitary motion of cells which are both stimulated or inhibited. Sherrington placed that reflexes need included activation and determined out reciprocal innervation of muscles through his research, which earned him the Nobel Prize. Sherrington moreover labored with Thomas Graham Brown, who furnished the imperative sample generator idea in 1911. Brown located out that the spinal cord may also form the essential stepping pattern with out the need for descending alerts from the brain. Their studies has had a incredible impact on our expertise of the way the aggravating device regulates motion.

Acetylcholine changed into the number one neurotransmitter decided inside the early 20th century. Henry Hallett Dale located it in 1915 for its effects on cardiac tissue. Otto Loewi mounted that acetylcholine changed into a neurotransmitter some years later, in 1921. Loewi proven its results on coronary coronary heart rate via demonstrating that a chemical secreted with the resource of the vagus nerve should reduce the heart rate of frogs. Since it have become secreted through the vagus nerve, Loewi termed it Vagusstoff. Loewi in the end determined that the Sympathicus Stuff, a chemical produced with the useful resource of manner of the sympathetic traumatic machine, come to be certainly adrenaline. This finding paved the manner for subsequent have a observe into neurotransmitters and their abilties inside the involved gadget.

Understanding the frame form of nerve impulses emerge as one of the most urgent problems for neuroscientists in the early 20th century. Between 1902 and 1912, Julius Bernstein made huge contributions to this issue with the aid of arguing that the motion functionality changed into as a result of a trade in the permeability of the axonal membrane to ions. He additionally advanced the Nernst equation for calculating resting potential throughout a membrane. In 1907, Louis Lapicque proposed that passing a threshold was the important element in growing an movement ability, which modified into later examined to be a quit result of ionic conductance dynamical systems.

Keith Lucas, a British physiologist, and his scholar Edgar Adrian had been inquisitive about the characteristic of sensory organs and nerve cells. In the primary decade of the twentieth century, Keith Lucas completed research that hooked up the all-or-nothing principle: muscle organizations both settlement certainly or in no manner. These discoveries have been noteworthy due to the fact they determined out that nerve impulses have been required for the aggravating device to originate and transmit messages.

With his direct observations of nerve fibers in motion, British physiologist Edgar Adrian modified the test of the neurological device. This approach enabled a broader form of checks and a latest diploma of precision in neurophysiology. Adrian's paintings has advocated technological tendencies required for undertaking anxious device studies. Adrian's early have a have a study turned into largely impacted by means of the usage of way of his investigations of processes vacuum tubes intercepted and amplified coded signals, similarly to his firsthand observations. Adrian's experiments substantially helped to our information of the manner neurons engage with each other.

Kenneth Cole made widespread contributions to neurophysiology sooner or later of his career at Columbia University in the mid-twentieth century. Cole's studies centered on simulating the electric tendencies of nerve tissue, and he collaborated with Howard Curtis to confirm Julius Bernstein's motion capability idea. Their findings display that membrane conductance rises during an motion capability. Around this time, David E. Goldman collaborated with Cole, and the Goldman equation have become advanced collectively in 1943. Alan Lloyd Hodgkin joined Cole at the Rockefeller Institute in 1937-38 to test the DC resistance of the membrane of the squid large axon in resting scenario. Cole and Hodgkin commenced out studying membrane potentials with internal electrodes within the big nerve fiber of the squid in 1939, prompting Cole to create the voltage clamp approach in 1947. These technological and conceptual advances paved the direction for future discoveries inside the discipline of neuroscience. A new age of neuroscience emerged within the mid-20th century,

23

focused on biochemistry and quantitative modeling of neuronal hobby. Bernard Katz became a pioneer on this situation, installing a model for synaptic neurotransmission in 1962. Beginning in 1966, Eric Kandel and his colleagues researched biochemical changes in neurons related to studying and reminiscence garage in the sea slug Aplysia. Their efforts culminated inside the Morris-Lecar model, superior in 1981 via Catherine Morris and Harold Lecar, which included the findings of Katz and Kandel's take a look at. These models laid the course for destiny advances in organic neuron models and neural computation models, ushering in a present day era of accuracy in thoughts research.

Many huge people finished pivotal contributions in establishing neurology as a amazing and cohesive situation within the mid-twentieth century. Among those credited with growing the sector as we understand it now encompass David Rioch, Francis O. Schmitt, and Stephen Kuffler. At the Walter Reed Army Institute of Research, Rioch pioneered the merging of anatomical and physiological research with scientific psychiatry. Schmitt, instead, based a neuroscience studies software program at the Massachusetts Institute of Technology that added together biology, chemistry, physics, and arithmetic. Meanwhile, in 1964, James L. McGaugh installation the primary freestanding neuroscience department (then referred to as Psychobiology) at the University of California, Irvine. Kuffler established the Department of Neurobiology at Harvard Medical School in 1966. It's in reality absolutely worth mentioning that the word "Neuroscience" can also had been coined for the number one time in 1962, whilst Schmitt installation his "Neuroscience Research Program" at MIT. These advances and partnerships helped to installation neuroscience as a separate location of study inside the later half of of of the 20 th century.

The observe of the thoughts has lengthy beyond through severa tiers in the route of statistics, which encompass philosophical, experimental, and theoretical degrees. Brain simulation is expected to play a critical position in furthering our expertise of this complicated organ within the destiny. Our information of the mind is now unmatched, and it is growing in tandem with new discoveries and technological breakthroughs.

Nevertheless, on the subject of how the mind abilties, one difficulty stays: Is it possible for humans to trade their private minds? In wonderful words, whilst we have completed developing and developing, can the thoughts go along with the float, adapt, and develop? This question takes us to the second one a part of this ebook, which examines the history of neuroplasticity.

Chapter 2: Neuroplasticity: Finding And Investigating

Sarah and Chris, neuroscientists at University College London's Spiers Lab, are conducting a chain of studies on James, the veteran London Taxi reason strain said in the ebook's organising.

Researchers are analyzing the brains of professional wayfinders to better apprehend how our brains adapt and exchange. They are specially appearing an intensive evaluation of taxi drivers' hippocampus, which has in no way been executed in advance than. They are mastering approximately how this location of the brain grows and matures in the course of time via analyzing the mouse hippocampus. The duties assigned to the taxi drivers are just like the navigational boundaries they confront on a every day basis, giving huge data approximately how the mind translates spatial records.

So wait, what precisely is a wayfinder? Neuroscientists use the term "wayfinding" to present an explanation for the complicated method via using manner of which our brains orient themselves in the worldwide. We utilize landmarks we recognize round us to get right of entry to a intellectual map of the surroundings primarily based on our previous evaluations. As we stated at the begin of this ebook, which will bypass The Knowledge and qualify for the interest, taxi drivers in London should be international-renowned wayfinders, which means that that remembering over 25,000 street names and information how to plan the most direct path between any two net sites within the metropolis.

James is now quietly secured into an MRI scanner. He's been there earlier than. Chris returns to the following-door place of job with Sarah after ensuring James is comfortable and sliding at the moving mattress into the extraordinary system. They press keys on their laptops to put together the MRI for its subsequent challenge.

Chris moves nearer, talking over his table microphone, that's associated with audio system in the MRI checking out room. "So, the following test we're going to do is a truly interesting test for us," he explains. "This is a immoderate-resolution image of your hippocampus. Do you want to begin?"

When James responds, a bit speaker at the table crackles to life. "Whenever you are organized."

"All good enough, it in reality is notable."

They enter a few greater commands. The MRI device hums because it powers up inside the next room. "The pastime will restart in some seconds with a few extraordinary 15 routes," Chris publicizes over the intercom.

"Okay."

Sarah is maintaining a list of routes within the the front of her. She answers the intercom and gives her London addresses. As Chris claims he has a plan, they begin asking him questions like, "Would you take road X?"

Chris considers his alternatives and responds with a sincere "positive" or "no." Sarah takes a one-of-a-type course after some questions and begins with a smooth set of sure-or-no questions.

Jimmy boldly answers the questions. This became what he'd been doing for the past many years. He is aware of his manner around London like the again of his hand. Meanwhile, Chris snap shots James's thoughts to illustrate how his mind reacts to the examination.

As we cited previously inside the e-book, London cab drivers have turn out to be a image of man or woman neuroplasticity, specifically within the hippocampal place of the mind. This area is maximum of the number one to thoughts impacted through Alzheimer's disease, and by way of learning the mouse hippocampus's increase styles, we're hoping to glean insights about its development in advance than its deterioration starts offevolved.

We can gather a better information of the hippocampus and its affiliation to Alzheimer's illness thru manner of reading its development in London cab drivers. Moreover, we can also discover if this individual adaptability and growth due to gaining The Knowledge and being a cab driving strain can provide a defensive trouble in opposition to the contamination. While these problems stay unsolved, analyzing skilled wayfinders and the changes of their brains can deliver essential insight into man or woman plasticity's potential for cognitive protection.

Of route, we have been aware of neuroplasticity lengthy earlier than we began discovering London taxi drivers. Part Two will take us back to the early 1900s to hint the evolution of our expertise of mind plasticity. We'll additionally see how neuroplasticity has become an critical element of our knowledge of the thoughts in cutting-edge years.

Defining Neuroplasticity

Nevertheless, before we circulate any farther, we first define neuroplasticity.

The word "neuroplasticity" refers to the mind's herbal ability to conform and redecorate itself with the beneficial aid of developing new neural connections and converting present ones. This basically manner that the mind can be rewired to feature in any other way than it did previously through the development and restructuring of its neural networks.

Neuroplasticity, additionally known as neural plasticity or thoughts plasticity, refers back to the mind's neural networks' tremendous capability to comply and alter through increase and rearrangement. Neuroplasticity reasons a wide type of changes, from the formation of new connections amongst person neuron circuits to extra fundamental alterations collectively with cortical remapping. Neuroplasticity offers itself in a mess of strategies, ranging from changes in circuits and networks due to studying a brand new potential or competence to the effect of outside variables which encompass environmental impacts, education, and mental stress.

Neuroplasticity modified into lengthy idea to be limited to infancy, but clinical research within the second half of of of the 20th century tested that the mind may additionally moreover additionally adjust or show plasticity during maturity. Yet, it's miles essential to spotlight that the growing thoughts is greater malleable than the person brain. Activity-set up plasticity is critical for wholesome improvement, learning, memory, and mind harm restoration.

The History of the Idea of Brain Plasticity

The belief of thoughts plasticity is often seen as a cutting-edge locating within the subject of neuroscience. Yet, the origins of this idea may be traced decrease lower returned to the past due 18th century. In 1793, Italian anatomist Michele Vicenzo Malacarne completed one of the first investigations on neuroplasticity. He paired animals, spent years education one of the pair, and then dissected each. Malacarne decided that the cerebellums of professional animals had been lots larger than those of untrained animals thru his observations.

Despite the importance of his discoveries, they were finally forgotten. Malacarne's discovery, however, lay the framework for the test of mind plasticity and set the manner for destiny discoveries in this thrilling scenario.

William James provided the concept that the mind and its characteristic had been no longer constant in stone and may exchange over time in his ebook The Principles of Psychology, published in 1890, however this idea come to be in particular omitted. James used the time period "plasticity" in 1890 to provide an reason behind a form that may be altered however no longer virtually transformed. Before the 1970s, however, professionals in neuroscience idea that the form and function of the thoughts have been regular and irreversible past adulthood.

It grow to be usually assumed within the early 1900s that the thoughts modified right into a nonrenewable organ. Yet, the word neuronal plasticity come to be utilized by the founder of neuroscience, Santiago Ramón y Cajal, to represent non pathological adjustments in the form of grownup brains. Cajal's neuron doctrine, which characterised the neuron because of the reality the fundamental unit of the involved system, laid the foundation for the belief of neural plasticity to emerge.

Santiago Ramón y Cajal used the time period "plasticity" to symbolize non-pathological modifications in brain shape in his work on degeneration and regeneration in person human beings' essential nervous structures. This end up in evaluation to the considerably held belief inside the early 1900s that the mind become a nonrenewable organ. Cajal's seminal neuron doctrine, which identified the neuron because of the reality the important unit of the stressful device, laid the inspiration for the concept of neural plasticity. Despite the reality that the time period "plasticity" have emerge as drastically used to symbolize the regeneration capability of the peripheral worried machine at the time, Cajal's software of the idea to the primary involved device aroused debate amongst positive neuroscientists.

Therefore, how could we come to recognize the plasticity of the mind? In the next element, we will check how research helped form this phrase into what it is now.

Neural Plasticity Research

In 1923, neurologist Karl Lashley carried out tests on rhesus monkeys that established changes in neural circuits and gave proof of plasticity. Although this massive discovery and specific records pointing to neuroplasticity, neuroscientists on the time did now not universally get hold of the belief.

Jerzy Konorski, a Polish neurophysiologist, made vital contributions to the sector of neurophysiology. He advanced secondary conditioned reflexes and operant conditioning, which extended our facts of methods the thoughts learns and adapts, based on Ivan Pavlov's studies. Konorski is also diagnosed for suggesting gnostic neurons, which might be just like the grandmother mobile hypothesis. Furthermore, he is credited with coining the word "neural plasticity," and he created theoretical theories approximately it that had been later provided thru Donald Hebb.

Jerzy Konorski based totally definitely a laboratory at the Nencki Institute of Experimental Biology together with his spouse, Liliana Lubinska, a neurophysiologist who earned her PhD beneath Louis Lapicque. Konorski's knowledge of neurophysiology extended because of Lubinskas facts, and he modified his interest to knowledge the neurological mechanics of conditioning. He made essential contributions to the subject, which incorporates discovering secondary conditioned reflexes and operant conditioning, as well as the idea of gnostic neurons, it genuinely is akin to the idea of grandmother cells. Konorski is also credited for coining the word "neural plasticity" and generating theoretical theories on the situation that have been much like Donald Hebb's.

Jerzy Konorski offered a vital task in his research of the neurological principles at the back of conditioning: how may conditioning modify the pre-current-day connections amongst neurons inside the thoughts? He provided a speculation similar to Donald Hebb's, which claims that unintended activation in time transforms ability connections into actual excitatory connections. Konorski went immediately to provide an motive in the back of that inhibitory connections form even as the stimulation of 1 enter is discovered by using manner of a reduction in its associated connection. This dynamic transformation, in step with Konorski, occurs through the improvement and proliferation of latest synaptic connections the diverse axon terminals of one nerve cellular and the soma (i.E., the frame and dendrites) of the possibility. Curiously, Donald Hebb one at a time articulated this comparable perception of synapse strengthening with utilization in his principle of Hebbian synapses in the West.

Justo Gonzalo decided in 1945 that the imperative cortex mass, which is located between the seen, tactile, and auditory projection areas, has plasticity competencies and the functionality to beautify neuronal excitability and rearrange pastime. Gonzalo saw this in some of thoughts damage sufferers, extensively those associated with inverted perception issues. He located that sensory inputs in the projection regions were in fact confined outlines that might be enlarged within the recruited cerebral mass and re-inverted in greater giant places through mind plasticity. Adaptation was established in the Stratton check, wherein people wore reversing glasses to appearance upright. Gonzalo's studies confirmed that the mind's center cortical mass modified into multimodal and will adjust to adjustments in belief dynamically.

From the second 1/2 of the 20 th century until the triumphing

Marian Cleeves Diamond end up a pioneer of contemporary neuroscience and an American scientist and educator. Her institution have become the primary to publish records indicating that the brain can exchange and expand with enjoy and enrichment, a concept known as neuroplasticity. Significantly, her studies on Albert Einstein's mind aided within the medical revolution in our expertise of the position of glial cells within the mind. Diamond's research as a professor of anatomy on the University of California, Berkeley, included the versions inside the cerebral cortex of male and girl rats, the connection amongst effective wondering and immunological health, and the illustration of girls in technology. In addition, her Integrative Biology lectures on YouTube were the arena's 2d most well-known college path in 2010.

Marian Diamond, a University of California, Berkeley researcher, became a number of the primary to offer medical proof of mind anatomical plasticity, which she published in 1964. Additional crucial statistics assisting the concept of neuroplasticity became generated in the Sixties and beyond, with noteworthy contributions from scientists which incorporates Paul Bach-y-Rita, Michael Merzenich, and Jon Kaas, among others.

Paul Bach-y-Rita, a neurologist from the Sixties, invented a machine that transformed visuals into vibrations that the customer felt via nubs inserted in a chair. Those with visible loss might also use this device to simulate vision via sensory substitution. Studies on stroke healing supplied more proof for the idea of neuroplasticity, demonstrating that wholesome mind regions may additionally additionally every now and then atone for the lack of competencies in damaged areas. Shepherd Ivory Franz made contributions to this field of examine.

Returning to the e-book's commencing, Eleanor Maguire discovered out that acquiring The Knowledge of London's Streets led to adjustments inside the shape of the hippocampus in taxi drivers. Maguire determined signs of gray depend redistribution in London taxi drivers as compared to controls, supplying insights into the plasticity of the hippocampus. This paintings piqued the curiosity of each the scientific network and the overall public, and it changed into extensively protected via the media worldwide.

Neuroplasticity: A Contemporary Perspective

Michael Merzenich is a trailblazing neuroscientist who has encouraged for neuroplasticity for over 3 a long term. He has made audacious claims within the career, claiming that brain exercise physical games can be as a achievement as medicinal capsules in treating excessive troubles along side schizophrenia. His findings suggest that the mind can adapt and modify inside the route of a person's life, even in antique age. Merzenich believes that even most of the aged, primary will increase in cognitive functioning, along with reading, notion, and reminiscence, are feasible. His research contradicts traditional know-how approximately brain getting old and opens up new avenues for cognitive development.

The innovative artwork of David Hubel and Torsten Wiesel, who tested kittens through stitching one eye near and reading cortical brain maps, impacted influential neurologist Michael Merzenich's research. They determined a few element unexpected: the brain area associated with close-eye come to be not inactive, but instead processed visible enter from the open eye. The mind appears to have determined a mechanism to set up itself as a way to maximize available cortical place.

Michael Merzenich have become a neurologist who questioned the significantly held concept that neuroplasticity takes area handiest in kids. During his postdoctoral research with Clinton Woosley, he have become interested in character plasticity. They studied what happened inside the brain whilst a peripheral nerve come to be severed and later regenerated. Merzenich's initial sight of adult plasticity came from this take a look at.

Michael Merzenich and Clinton Woosley done a pioneering experiment in which they mapped the hand maps of monkey brains earlier than and after severing a peripheral nerve and sewing the ends together. The outcomes had been startling because of the truth the expectedly disordered hand map inside the mind was clearly normal. Merzenich came to the conclusion that the perception that people are born with a set, hardwired tool needed to be faulty. He contended that the mind needed to be malleable, with the functionality to accurate its form in response to aberrant enter. His observe on the techniques that permit revel in and neural interest to modify thoughts function furnished him the 2016 Kavli Prize in Neuroscience.

This belief of a thoughts that could adapt and adjust dynamically in response to activities is charming, however how does it have an effect on us in recent times? Several hypotheses have emerged in brand new years on how we may additionally moreover rent neuroplasticity standards to higher our lives and deal with trauma. Part Three is probably devoted to this concern.

Chapter 3: Brain Plasticity's Uses

Every discovery has ramifications that aren't constantly obvious. Many of the scientists indexed within the preceding section may not have realized how the mind can rewire itself, repair itself, and enlarge in sudden strategies. Such findings may also additionally furthermore have modified the manner we look at and perform these days.

Without a doubt, information mind plasticity has medical advantages. Chris and Sarah, who've a have a look at the brains of London taxi drivers, take shipping of as proper with that their research will result in drug remedies that might save you Alzheimer's and other nerve or mind problems. But, in this final segment, we will cope with mind programs.

Alzheimer's illness and other nerve or mind ailments. But, on this ultimate phase, we are capable of cognizance on applications of mind plasticity that we're capable of all use in our every day lives. We'll start with self-education through looking at the work of Hani Akasheh, a younger guy.

Brain Education and Hani Akasheh

Hani Akasheh became born in Jordan and learnt the importance and uses of neuroplasticity within the path of his adolescence. "My brother and I grew up in an irritating own family, with a mom who had a predisposition for persistent depression and tension and a father who became emotionally remote," Hani explains. As a give up stop result, no matter the fact that Hani went on to turn out to be a doctor and his brother an engineer, each of them had highbrow illnesses same to their mom's. Hani struggled with tension and depression as a more youthful guy, which caused him to pursue a career in psychiatry.

Hani and his brother, now grownups, began chatting about how the mind works. This brought about an exciting discovery. "It's humorous how one element we learnt approximately how our thoughts works, knowledge how our mind works," he says.

"It intrigues me that one essential notion in neuroscience has the functionality, capacity, and promise to decorate and remodel people's highbrow fitness," he goes on to say. "This vital concept is referred to as mind plasticity. It's referred to as neuroplasticity in my concern."

Hani claims that virtually reading approximately mind plasticity, or the concept that the mind can remodel and reorganize itself, helped him address his tension and despair better. This finding recommended the 2 brothers to move back to Jordan in order to assist those tormented by intellectual and emotional illnesses. The idea become to educate people "crucial neuroscience standards that we felt may additionally moreover assist them transform their outlook on highbrow fitness," as Hani places it.

"We combined seen animations and technology to increase a fun and exciting technique for people to investigate greater approximately their brains, and we had been simply fortunate and relatively completely satisfied to look our agency make bigger so fast on this form of short time period. Engaging with humans from all walks of existence, schools, IT businesses, and enterprise behemoths." So, what changed into the prevent give up stop end result? Educating human beings from all areas of lifestyles and supporting them in converting their wondering.

Changing the manner humans perception altered the wiring of their mind.

Simply located, Hani and his brother have been training people a manner to out-expect melancholy via the use of harnessing the maximum modern-day thoughts plasticity breakthroughs. "When we placed out this idea, and we reached out to adults laid low with stress and anxiety, and we recommended them approximately mind plasticity and the relationship the various frontal cortex and the amygdala, the strength of the message itself gave them intrinsic motivation to understand how powerful meditation and mindfulness may be in controlling your anxiety and pressure signs and symptoms," Hani keeps.

Years later, Hani and his brother have once more to Jordan for a second time, this time to teach kindergarten teachers approximately neuroplasticity. Teachers that have this facts can help their younger university college students understand that they will be able to in reality adjust their lives truely via changing their standpoint on life. According to research, a toddler's style of wondering, their mindset on life, and their self-photo have a massive impact on the relaxation in their lives.

What about us? We can also find out the electricity of incredible and exquisite questioning in truth with the useful resource of information how the mind adapts and evolves. We learn how to shift our perspectives, which impacts the shape and density of our future brains.

To Alter The Brain, Kelly Lambert and Physical Behaviors

Dr. Kelly Lambert contends that enhancing your actions and surroundings can virtually improve your neuroplasticity. She also believes that this will result in a far more powerful treatment for melancholy than a medicine.

One incredible advantage of neuroplasticity is its capability to help us in adapting to new and disturbing settings. Individuals with greater brain plasticity are an awful lot much less disturbing even as faced with new troubles. Yet, how do you increase your neuroplasticity?

Lambert's research with lab rats showed that physical conduct had a large effect on thoughts plasticity. She factors out, for example, that the high-quality majority of neurons in our brains are without delay tied to bodily movement. "People want to assume that the mind is for wondering, however it's really extra for movement than wondering," she explains.

When we hold in thoughts this facts, we might also additionally infer that the current-day lifestyle of sitting about and viewing monitors for every artwork and pleasure has a awful effect on our brains, probably contributing to increased disappointment in our society. What can be the solution if this had been the case? Increased physical hobby.

Lambert separated the lab rats into companies. For example, one enterprise of rats became virtually given food and rewards and were now not required to paintings for them. A second group of rats needed to "acquire" food thru digging for it in hay hundreds. After many weeks, each rats were introduced to a contemporary surroundings— water. Because that they have got been grown in a lab, neither set of rats had ever visible a big body of water. What would possibly their reaction be?

The rats used to tough paintings physically for his or her food have been a long manner extra ambitious, diving into the water with very little fear. The rats that had in no way needed to hard work have been hectic at the sight of water and took notably longer to regulate to their new environment.

What is the takeaway? Lambert determined that the rats who worked had rewired their brains at the same time as she tested the brains of each organizations of rats. They'd positioned the hard way that difficult try and innovation paid off. Their brains had been validated to be greater pliable than those of folks who had in no manner needed to difficult paintings.

We may additionally consequently make our brains greater malleable and adaptable through wearing out any bodily activity that offers pleasure, collectively with knitting, cooking, building something, or gardening.

Physical paintings, like rats, can help us face new situations with an awful lot much less tension and fear.

Meditation And Neuroplasticity

Meditation changed into as soon as considered a horrible time period in Western society. The tremendous people who pondered had been hippies who significantly utilized lax morals and some of recreational capsules. Because of this stigma, few researchers took meditation extensively until in recent times.

Scientists have scanned the brains of life-prolonged meditators and decided that ordinary practice of meditation reduces anxiety, avoids persistent despair, and enhances relationships, compassion, and fashionable highbrow and emotional properly-being. This is because of the fact that the brain areas responsible for such abilities are substantially thicker in experienced meditators than in others.

How can we use this data? It facilitates the discoveries made at some degree in the e-book. We can also additionally hire practices like meditation and yoga to modify our brains, preparing our minds to deal with strain and confront the world with peace and composure, way to the plasticity of the brain.

Understanding how the thoughts works—and the way it is able to modify itself through the years, as we've got seen in some examples—ought to have a big effect on how we confront the future. It has been mounted that truly understanding that our brains are changeable improves our defenses in competition to tension and depression. Nevertheless, at the same time as we learn how to use our everyday practices to influence how our brains boom—as an instance, thru physical physical sports and meditation—we empower ourselves to satisfy new situations and problems with calm, compassion, and creativity.

Chapter 4: Rewiring Your Brain

The state of affairs of neuroscience has made high-quality improvement in today's years, revolutionizing our information of the human mind. In the beyond, it changed into believed that the mind we were born with become the identical mind we would have for the rest of our lives and that our genes in large part decided our thoughts, feelings, and movements. However, modern-day discoveries in neuroscience have tested that the thoughts is a long way greater malleable than formerly believed and that our studies and moves can profoundly effect how our brains are burdened out.

Neuroplasticity is one of the maximum thrilling standards in neuroscience, which refers to the mind's capacity to alternate and adapt in response to reviews. We now recognize that the thoughts can create new neural pathways and even generate new neurons for the duration of our lives, so we can maintain to analyze and develop nicely into adulthood. This starkly differs from the vintage view that the mind have emerge as in massive component regular and unchangeable after childhood.

Another key idea in neuroscience is neurogenesis, which refers back to the thoughts's capability to generate new neurons. For a few years, it become believed that we have been born with a hard and fast quantity of neurons and could in no manner generate new ones. However, cutting-edge-day research have validated that the mind can generate new neurons in excessive quality areas, inclusive of the hippocampus, this is concerned in memory and gaining knowledge of. This shows that we are capable of actively decorate our mind function via way of task sports promoting neurogenesis, together with workout and gaining understanding of recent abilties.

Social systems are each other region of neuroscience that has received lots hobby in present day years. Mirror neurons, for instance, are specialized neurons that fireside even as we act and feature a have a look at a person else performing the identical movement. This indicates that our brains are stressed for empathy and social connection and that our social interactions have a powerful impact on how our brains are wired.

Nutritional neuroscience is every different rising location of studies that has shed slight on how weight loss plan may additionally have an effect on thoughts characteristic. For example, we now realize that fantastic nutrients, at the side of omega-three fatty acids, are critical for thoughts health and might assist to prevent cognitive decline. Similarly, a weight-reduction plan immoderate in sugar and processed meals has been associated with various cognitive and emotional problems.

By information the ones thoughts and making use of them to our lives, we are capable of take manage of our thoughts fitness and improve our well-being. For example, reading to be calm and exquisite can profoundly effect how our brains are careworn out. By running towards mindfulness, meditation, and distinctive rest techniques, we are capable of reduce stress and anxiety, which can help rewire our brains for added resilience and emotional regulation.

In this book, we are capable of discover the way to use the current-day findings in neuroscience to make the maximum of our strengths and overcome our weaknesses. We will communicate sensible techniques for boosting reminiscence, building relationships, and snoozing nicely. By making those adjustments, we will rewire our brains to be calmer, happier, and extra resilient in facing existence's worrying situations.

Moving Away from Nature vs. Nurture

The human brain is a complex and first-rate organ that weighs splendid 3 kilos however has many abilties that manage every detail of our being. Understanding how the thoughts works is essential to rewiring it and improving our cognitive and emotional properly-being.

The thoughts interacts with the outdoor worldwide, and our stories drastically shape our nature. It is broadly commonplace that nature and nurture aren't opposing forces however paintings together to influence our person, conduct, and cognitive capabilities.

The brain is tender-wired, now not hardwired, due to this it can adapt and alternate in the course of existence. Unlike a laptop chip that has a hard and fast layout, the mind is malleable and may be rewired through gaining knowledge of, experience, and high-quality interventions. Brain plasticity, the capability to exchange neural pathways and connections, is at the center of rewiring the mind. By records how the thoughts is prepared and methods facts, we're capable of harness the power of plasticity to enhance our cognitive and emotional functioning.

The mind consists of about one hundred billion neurons and lots of different cells that artwork collectively to control our thoughts, emotions, and conduct. Neurons are specialized cells that speak with every extraordinary via electric powered powered and chemical alerts. These cells are grouped into modules, which include the cortex, this is the thoughts's outer layer and has hemispheres, four lobes, and subcortical modules beneath the cortex.

The right and left hemispheres of the mind have extremely good capabilities, in spite of the truth that they artwork collectively to technique facts. The right hemisphere processes seen and spatial facts, permitting us to appearance the massive photograph and understand styles. It is also associated with feelings, creativity, and intuition. The left hemisphere, but, is worried in processing language, common feel, and analytical wondering. It is better at organizing facts and records linearly, together with in writing or mathematics.

The corpus callosum is a band of fibers connecting the brain's hemispheres. It lets in the 2 components of the mind to speak and work together to method information. Research indicates that girls have a thicker corpus callosum than guys, because of this that the 2 facets of their brains speak higher, ensuing in a more balanced mind. Conversely, guys have an asymmetrical torque, with the proper frontal lobe and left occipital lobe being greater outstanding.

The thoughts's proper hemisphere is greater emotional and has higher connections with the elements of the thoughts beneath the cortex. This location is answerable for empathy, instinct, and social cognition. Women are considered more intuitive than guys due to the fact their brains have better connections the various aspects, giving phrases more emotional this means that. They additionally have a tendency to be more empathic, that is the capacity to apprehend and percentage the feelings of others.

The mind's left hemisphere is more worried in language processing, inclusive of talking, writing, and analyzing. It is higher at processing statistics linearly and sequentially, and this area is likewise involved in not unusual experience, reasoning, and trouble-solving. The left hemisphere takes over as soon as a few trouble is well-known, at the equal time as the right factor is greater active whilst mastering a few factor new.

The mind is divided into 4 lobes: the frontal lobe, middle (parietal) lobe, factor (temporal) lobe, and again (occipital) lobe, every with its particular abilties. When you need something, which includes a chair, your mind strategies numerous factors of it during specific lobes. For example, your right parietal lobe stores the chair's form, your left temporal lobe recollects the terms your friend used to provide an reason for their Costa Rica journey, and your right temporal lobe recalls the tone of their voice. The occipital lobe recalls the chair's shade as you go away the room.

Women have more neurons inside the part of the brain chargeable for language, giving them a bonus in verbal conversation. This is obvious from the age of while women start speaking six months in advance than boys. When building verbal plans, women rely greater on the left hippocampus, at the identical time as men excel in seen and spatial skills because of the better activity inside the proper hippocampus.

The maximum present day part of evolution is the frontal lobe, comprising 20% of the human thoughts. In assessment, a cat's frontal lobe occupies best 3.Five% of its mind. The prefrontal cortex (PFC), located on the the the the front of the frontal lobe, is answerable for complex cognitive, emotional, and behavioral abilities. It allows humans to create a moral code and prioritize others' dreams over their personal. Damage to the PFC outcomes in impulsive conduct and hurting others.

The dorsolateral prefrontal cortex (DLPFC) is vital for better-diploma thinking, short-term reminiscence, and hobby. It is the final part of the thoughts to mature and the primary to weaken with age. In evaluation, the orbital frontal cortex (OFC) develops early in life and is connected to feelings and social cognition. A damaged OFC, like that of Phineas Gage, can result in impulsivity and issue controlling feelings.

The OFC is critical for retaining close to relationships and regulating emotions, and it stays steady as one age and lets in clean take into account of faces. Finally, the left and proper prefrontal cortices have distinct features, with the proper PFC assisting in foresight and famous making plans and the left PFC helping with interest to element.

Unlocking the Secrets of Complex Relationship Between Neurons and Their Messengers

Billions of neurons art work together inside the mind, forming complicated networks that permit us to assume, enjoy, and bypass. These neurons are positioned in extremely good mind areas, with each region answerable for unique functions.

In every location of the mind, neurons paintings together, forming connections and speakme through neurotransmitters. These neurotransmitters are crucial for the brain's characteristic, wearing messages throughout tiny gaps known as synapses. There are many one among a kind types of neurotransmitters, each with its specific position in thoughts characteristic.

One of the most important neurotransmitters is glutamate, an excitatory neurotransmitter that allows set off neurons and reason diverse mind features. Glutamate consists of many methods, collectively with learning, memory, movement, and belief.

Another essential neurotransmitter is gamma-aminobutyric acid (GABA), an inhibitory neurotransmitter that slows down thoughts interest and promotes calmness. GABA regulates anxiety, mood, and sleep, and drugs like Valium and Ativan are designed to enhance their effects.

Neurons are distinctly adaptable and may alternate their connections and abilties over time. This adaptability, referred to as neuroplasticity, permits the thoughts to rewire itself in reaction to new opinions and mastering. For example, if you look at a ultra-modern language or expand a state-of-the-art potential, neurons in the corresponding location of the thoughts will form new connections and guide cutting-edge ones, allowing you to perform the challenge greater efficiently over the years.

In addition to glutamate and GABA, many special neurotransmitters play essential roles in thoughts characteristic. These neurotransmitters may also moreover furthermore only make up a small fraction of the interactions among neurons, but they could significantly have an effect on neuronal interest. As a end result, they were the state of affairs of sizeable studies, and lots of pills had been advanced to goal them.

Among those neurotransmitters, serotonin, norepinephrine, and dopamine are some of the most considerably studied. They are referred to as neuromodulators because of the reality they are capable of alter the sensitivity of receptors, enhance neuronal interest, or stimulate glutamate production. Additionally, they could help clean out unwanted signals in the brain thru way of blockading them from engaging in the synapse, even though in some cases, they can also boom different signs. Like glutamate and GABA, those neurotransmitters can act straight away or adjust the glide of data through the synapses.

Serotonin has acquired masses interest because of the big use of medication like Prozac. Serotonin performs a essential function in regulating our feelings and temper. Low serotonin ranges were related to tension, despair, or even obsessive-compulsive ailment (OCD).

Serotonin may be taken into consideration a shape of police officer inside the thoughts, supporting to maintain hobby ranges in check. Individuals taking antidepressants like Prozac often report feeling less with the beneficial useful resource of factors that could commonly motive them distress. However, this effect can be a downside, as a few human beings may also moreover revel in emotionally numb or a notable deal less aware of immoderate fine memories on the identical time as taking those medicinal pills.

Other vital neurotransmitters within the thoughts encompass acetylcholine, histamine, and adenosine. Acetylcholine is important for learning and memory, and it's miles worried inside the control of muscle contractions. Alzheimer's sickness, characterised via reminiscence loss and cognitive decline, is connected to reduced acetylcholine levels. Drugs that growth acetylcholine degrees, like

Aricept, are used to deal with Alzheimer's illness.

Histamine is notion for its role inside the immune device and allergies, but it moreover performs an essential function within the mind. It regulates wakefulness and alertness; low histamine degrees are related to sleep problems like narcolepsy. Drugs that block histamine, like Benadryl, can purpose drowsiness.

Adenosine is involved in regulating sleep and wakefulness, and caffeine, a commonplace stimulant, works by using manner of manner of blockading adenosine receptors. When adenosine tiers are immoderate, we enjoy sleepy, however whilst caffeine blocks adenosine receptors, we sense more alert and conscious.

Understanding the neurotransmitters inside the mind and the way they art work is critical for developing new capsules to treat neurological and psychiatric issues. By centered on specific neurotransmitters, scientists can growth more powerful drugs with fewer factor effects. However, it's far critical to take into account that the mind is complex, and plenty of mysteries continue to be to be solved.

Synchronization of Neurons

Over the beyond a few years, research has examined that synapses are not everyday entities however continuously converting, called neuroplasticity or synaptic plasticity. The connections among neurons, known as synapses, are also venture to change. Neuroplasticity is crucial to reminiscence formation. When we studies some thing new, our mind alters the connections among nerve cells, permitting us to consider it. If the mind became static, new reading is probably not possible. When we set up connections among ideas or snap shots, we additionally installation connections some of the neurons that maintain them.

The concept of "Use it or lose it" applies to neuroplasticity. Synaptic connections that underpin a skill turn out to be more potent while we use them and weaker at the same time as we do not, much like muscle groups. "Cells that fire collectively twine collectively" is a beneficial way of explaining how the thoughts transforms whilst we examine a few aspect new. The connections amongst neurons that fireplace in unison at the same time as we carry out a particular motion or recall reminiscence grow to be more potent the extra we do it. The more regularly the neurons fireplace collectively, the greater the threat they may fire together once more.

The word "Cells that fireplace collectively twine together" has grow to be a considerably used announcing in neuroscience. However, a corresponding word says, "Neurons that fireplace aside cord apart," that means that neurons that do not synchronize cannot shape connections. This explains why we neglect subjects.

In essence, repetition is pinnacle to developing robust neural connections. For instance, athletes and musicians engage in ordinary workout training to enhance their skills. Similarly, the more we remember something, the greater regularly it involves mind. This repetition alters the wiring of the mind, principal to the formation of conduct.

The greater frequently neurons hearth together, the quicker they come to be, which enhances the thoughts's performance. For instance, on the equal time as we first learn how to ride a bike, we use more muscular tissues and neurons due to the fact we are wobbly. However, fewer neurons and muscle mass are required with exercising, major to smoother and faster rides. This takes area because of the truth the neurons have associated and advanced robust neural pathways.

As we enhance our skills, the thoughts creates extra place to cope with them. For instance, studies have confirmed that regular motion can increase neuroplasticity and create greater place in the thoughts. Alvaro Pascual-

Leone from Harvard Medical School used transcranial magnetic stimulation (TMS) to degree particular elements of the cortex. He decided that the reading palms of blind folks that take a look at Braille had big cortical maps than their different fingers and the palms of sighted readers. Essentially, their studying hands had emerge as so sensitive that they required greater place within the brain.

Neuroplasticity is a time period used to explain the mind's potential to alternate and adapt. The connections between neurons (synapses) may be reinforced or weakened via repeated use or lack thereof. The phrase "cells that fireside collectively cord collectively" describes how the mind adjustments while we research some element new. By repeating a project, the connections among activated neurons become stronger, making the task an awful lot much less complex to carry out.

Conversely, "neurons that fireplace apart twine aside" manner that neurons that aren't activated collectively will now not join. This is why we frequently forget about things we do not use or exercising regularly.

Practicing a ability time and again makes us better at that expertise and changes the way our brain is stressed. As we become greater gifted, the mind turns into greater green, the usage of fewer neurons to carry out the equal task. This is why professional musicians and athletes have greater location inside the mind committed to the specific factors of the frame they use most often.

Interestingly, highbrow exercising also can assist alternate how the thoughts works. Just imagining performing a venture can stimulate the identical neural pathways as bodily appearing the challenge. This technique that intellectual exercise by myself can enhance our skills and trade how the mind is forced out.

The Fascinating Science of Neuroplasticity

Long-term potentiation (LTP) is a phenomenon that takes vicinity even as cells remain excited for an prolonged duration. It strengthens connections among cells, developing the likelihood of them firing together in the future. LTP can remaining a long time and takes vicinity through converting the electrochemical connections among neurons. The component of the synapse that sends indicators, referred to as glutamate, will increase in garage, and the receiving component adjustments to really accept greater glutamate. Additionally, inside the resting united states, the voltage on the receptor factor strengthens, which attracts in more glutamate. If the neurons preserve firing, the genes inner might be activated, developing more building blocks for the infrastructure and further strengthening their courting.

Brain-derived neurotrophic trouble (BDNF) is a crucial protein for neuroplasticity and neurogenesis. BDNF enables to assemble, expand, and maintain the infrastructure of cellular circuitry, making it one of the most researched subjects in neuroscience. It works as a sort of fertilizer, main to the boom of cells even as applied to them. BDNF makes cells make bigger hastily, stimulating the growth of latest branches on neurons, much like the growth inside the mind while analyzing takes place.

BDNF works in numerous processes to sell neuroplasticity and neurogenesis:

1. It activates genes within the mobile that purpose more proteins, serotonin, and BDNF to be produced.

2. It sticks to the receptors on the synapse, growing a waft of ions that increases the voltage and strengthens connections amongst neurons. Overall, BDNF prevents cells from demise and allows them expand and stay healthy. It additionally circuitously turns on the production of antioxidants and protecting proteins by turning on glutamate.

3.   It promotes lengthy-time period potentiation, it's far essential for neuroplasticity.

LTP and BDNF are carefully associated, and learning will increase the quantity of BDNF in the brain. When BDNF isn't always gift, the thoughts can not carry out LTP. Not the use of neural connections outcomes in their weakening and eventual loss of life, at the identical time as the use of them makes them more potent. Long-time period depression (LTD) is a method that helps destroy lousy behavior and hyperlinks among neurons. LTD makes vintage connections weaker, liberating up more neurons that may be used to make new connections.

An instance of this principle is studying a contemporary language. If someone learns a extremely-modern-day language of their twenties, they may probably communicate it with a distinctive accent than their first language. However, if a person learns a second language at age nine, they'll probable no longer have any accessory from their first language. Adults generally generally generally tend to keep the neural connections that make particular sounds, even though attempting to research new sounds. The extra a person talks to folks that do not have an accessory, the much more likely their accent will go away.

Changes in the mind get up more rapid whilst new mind or insights are discovered out than whilst getting to know a cutting-edge language or losing an accent. Some components of the brain excel at rapid connecting statistics to make selections, and spindle cells are critical. These precise neurons be a part of one among a type types of records speedy and efficaciously within the cingulate cortex. Spindle cells permit for quick hassle-fixing and desire-making, even in immoderate-emotion situations.

However, spindle cells can't paintings in the occasion that they've little to do. The thoughts have to be prepared for rewiring with the resource of studying new subjects and growing new skills. Neural networks which have already been created are used to gather statistics and form new connections, main to the technology of latest thoughts and the capacity to make quick selections.

How We Make Quick Decisions?

A precise type of nerve cell known as spindle cell is noticeably responsive and is enough inside the human thoughts in assessment to unique species. It is speculated that this abundance of spindle cells is one of the reasons why people are able to making snap options. These cells are characterized via their bulbous give up and lengthy, thick extension and are about four instances large than specific neurons, making them first-class for fast communique within the mind.

Spindle cells play a essential characteristic in social relationships, emotions, and remedy because of the reality they are placed in the mind and connect to one-of-a-kind components of the social mind. They have a immoderate density of synaptic receptors for dopamine, serotonin, and vasopressin, all recognized to effect mood and emotional states. Spindle cells facilitate connections some of the OFC and the cingulate cortex, with loads of these cells located within the frontal region of the cingulate cortex. These cells are important for establishing bonds and helping in social communique.

Imagine you are making plans a holiday to New Orleans, however at the manner, you listen at the radio that Hurricane Katrina is coming close to close to. Your spindle cells act, and also you fast exchange your direction to Houston. Upon arriving in Houston, you observe that many Katrina refugees were relocated to the Astrodome, and also you spend part of your tour volunteering at a nearby soup kitchen. These impromptu selections in complex conditions significantly impacted human beings's feelings, and you could remember this adventure as one in every of your maximum cherished recollections within the destiny years.

As you revisit this tale, the statistics you bear in mind will determine which synapses to your thoughts grow to be stronger or weaker. Additionally, as you share this tale with others, the story also can trade, causing your thoughts to modify as well. Your buddies may additionally moreover furthermore percentage their reviews on the authorities's reaction, linking your recollections and emotions.

Two thoughts systems, the amygdala, and hippocampus, are liable for our capacity to recall sports activities. The amygdala, shaped like an almond and taken from the Greek word for almond, "amygdalon," is activated with the useful resource of sturdy feelings inclusive of fear, giving each reminiscence an emotional depth. Whether it's far a glance from an appealing person or a stern gaze out of your boss, the amygdala acts as a panic button, triggering a reaction to the perceived chance.

The hippocampus derives its name from the Greek word for "seahorse," every different brain form concerned in memory retention. Recent studies have placed that neurogenesis, the technology of new neurons, can arise within the hippocampus, opposite to preceding beliefs. This new finding emphasizes the significance of working on reminiscence to rewire the mind.

The hippocampus and amygdala are chargeable for two sorts of reminiscence: specific and implicit. Explicit memory refers back to the recollect of statistics, dates, and terms, inclusive of remembering what you had for dinner remaining night time time or the name of a acquainted man or woman. Implicit reminiscence, however, is the unconscious reminiscence of emotional sports activities and situations. For instance, the fight-or-flight reaction is activated while a functionality risk is detected, even with out aware awareness.

This computerized reaction tool has been crucial for the survival of our ancestors, who needed to react speedy to danger with out wasting time on cognitive processing. The amygdala is a brief course to this response device, triggering the combat-or-flight response when vital.

The mind's frontal lobes are critical for selection-making, problem-solving, and making plans. They additionally play a essential function in regulating emotions and handling stress. When you're glad and engaged in sports activities that you enjoy, your frontal lobes are extra lively, that could definitely impact your regular mind feature.

On the opposite hand, continual strain and anxiety can harm your thoughts's government control center, leading to impaired desire-making, reminiscence, and emotional regulation. This is due to the fact chronic stress can cause changes inside the shape and feature of the thoughts, alongside aspect the prefrontal cortex, it's far a key a part of the frontal lobes.

Therefore, looking after your highbrow and emotional health is important thru carrying out sports that promote relaxation, together with meditation, mindfulness, and exercising. Doing so can help balance your sympathetic and parasympathetic concerned systems, decorate your mind feature, and decorate your commonplace well-being.

The OFC (orbitofrontal cortex) and distinctive mind components are known as the "social mind" due to the fact they're involved in social interactions and relationships. The excellent of your social connections could have an impact in your highbrow health and normal nicely-being. These neural connections are standard through the use of way of your relationships, beginning along with your mother and father as a infant and evolving all through your existence.

The neurochemical oxytocin plays a characteristic in bonding and social connection. It is occasionally called the "cuddle hormone" because it lets in lessen pain and boom first-rate emotions while interacting with others.

Mirror neurons are every exceptional crucial discovery in records social interactions and empathy. These neurons assist you to enjoy and recognize the emotions and moves of others without consciously thinking about them. For instance, while you see a person yawn, your reflect neurons might also cause you to revel in the urge to yawn.

The social thoughts is an essential part of our everyday mind function and properly-being, and wholesome social relationships can without a doubt effect our highbrow and bodily fitness.

This passage discusses the location of reflect neurons in social interactions, empathy, and compassion. It moreover explores the blessings of mindfulness meditation and prayer on mind feature and highbrow fitness.

The reflect neuron tool is critical in how people relate to themselves and others. Individuals with autism might also moreover have troubles with the replicate neuron machine, that could impact their capability to connect to others.

Feeling empathy and compassion via the reflect neuron system has been related to having compassion for oneself. Giving to others and being kind advantages intellectual fitness, while selfishness may be destructive.

Mindfulness meditation and prayer had been observed to trade the mind in great approaches. Studies have established that years of meditation can regulate thoughts artwork, main to better health and happiness. A conscious mind can be executed through meditation and help people exchange how their brains artwork.

Revamp Your Mind with the Powerful FEED Method

Now that you've higher understood how the thoughts operates allow's delve right into a manner to modify its functioning. The method we talk includes 4 steps called "FEED." John B. Arden first added it in his e-book "Rewire Your Brain." It is a extraordinary e-book to have a have a look at on Neuroplasticity. The approach includes the subsequent steps:

- Focus

- Effort

- Effortlessness

- Determination

The first step is to 'Focus.'

To exchange how your thoughts works, you have to recognize of the situation, behavior, or memory you need to maintain. This triggers the frontal lobes of your mind, which set off different factors of your mind. Consider this the alert characteristic. It's no longer feasible to modify the manner your mind features without starting off alternate. A plan is a extremely good way to start. Attention and the frontal lobes are vital additives of neuroplasticity. The PFC is just like the mind's brain, guiding sources to vital areas. If you are on autopilot, like driving and talking to a pal, you may undergo in mind the verbal exchange, no longer the environment. But in case you interest on what you see, your hobby will shift, and you'll preserve extra bodily data of the experience. Discussing those statistics later will aid in memory retention. You're a lot less likely to undergo in mind the ones info in case you do not have a have a look at them. Simply paying interest isn't always enough to adjust the way your mind capabilities. Your mind can not hold the whole lot with such a number of subjects vying on your hobby every day. Focus on the present 2nd is what triggers neuroplasticity.

The 2d step is to Make an Effort.

Focusing your strive on a venture shifts your hobby from statement to movement. This planned try turns on the thoughts to shape new connections among neurons. Learning some element new calls for a big quantity of glucose to gasoline thoughts hobby. In brand new a long time, researchers have made first rate discoveries about thoughts function through way of studying PET scans, illuminating the areas of the thoughts which might be lively within the route of particular duties or feelings. This interest is a prevent give up result of glucose metabolism inside the ones precise areas. Initial tries at a trendy mission will activate the corresponding region of the mind because it adapts to the goals of the hobby.

Chapter 5: Emotional Control

"The true hero is one that conquers his private anger and hatred."

Dalai Lama

Navigating the Difference Between Stress and False Alarms

Anxiety can be overwhelming, with fear being considered one in each of its critical culprits. When fear units in, it triggers an alarm that can motive plenty of symptoms, together with a racing coronary heart, shortness of breath, and immoderate fear. But what takes place while the alarm goes off, and there is no actual danger? That's what is referred to as a faux alarm. Learning a way to prevent faux alarms from going off is vital to correctly coping with tension.

To understand the way to do that, allow's begin with the amygdala, the a part of the mind responsible for fear. Ideally, the amygdala have to have a harmonious dating with the orbitofrontal cortex (OFC). For many human beings, this dating begins offevolved in youth and continues in some unspecified time in the future in their lives, thanks to exceptional and nurturing reports.

However, the amygdala can be overactive for others and act as a panic button for every real and fake alarms. This takes vicinity while the amygdala and OFC fail to talk well. In this situation, the OFC turns into useless, and tension signs and symptoms can increase. The specific records is that the OFC can help calm the amygdala and save you it from overreacting.

It's crucial to phrase which you do not need to shut down the amygdala completely; as an alternative, you want to "tame" it to work for you. Doing so makes you more attuned for your emotions, not actually fear. In brief, to govern anxiety correctly, it's far critical to discover ways to save you fake alarms from going off and to foster a wholesome dating among the amygdala and OFC.

The amygdala may be activated in number one ways: the slow song and the fast track. The slow music passes thru the cortex, which permits you to hold in thoughts matters earlier than fear gadgets in. This can be beneficial because of the fact you may rationalize and inform your self there can be now not anything to worry. However, it may also be damaging if you boom irrational fears.

On the opposite hand, the fast tune to activating the amygdala can reason a extra instant response. This triggers the sympathetic irritating machine, which can result in emotions of anxiety or panic. Before your cortex can approach what's happening, your amygdala can sound the alarm. In a fragment of a 2d, the amygdala uses norepinephrine to ship electric powered impulses via the sympathetic fearful tool, stimulating the adrenal glands to release epinephrine (adrenaline) into your bloodstream. This creates a jolt that will increase your breathing, coronary coronary heart charge, and blood stress, known as the fight-or-flight response.

The fight-or-flight reaction is a beneficial survival mechanism for all mammals within the wild. The first step is to freeze, it honestly is a way for animals to emerge as invisible and look at the situation earlier than figuring out to combat or flee. For instance, while using at night time time time on a rustic avenue and encountering a deer reputation inside the middle of the street, the deer will freeze to discover any functionality predators. Once it determines the predator's vicinity, it may keep with the rest of the combat-or-flight reaction, both through fighting or strolling away. Even even though it can appear to be the deer is doing no longer whatever, its body is getting ready to achieve this.

When confronted with a threat, the frame's natural response activates the combat-or-flight reaction, which prepares the frame to fight or flee the chance. The amygdala initiates this reaction, which sends signs to the hypothalamus, the part of the autonomic worried machine that regulates many metabolic procedures.

There are ways wherein the amygdala may be activated: the sluggish track, which passes through the cortex and allows for rational idea earlier than the feeling of worry sets in, and the quick tune, which bypasses the cortex and triggers a proper away reaction. This on the spot response sets off the sympathetic worried tool and releases adrenaline and cortisol from the adrenal glands.

Adrenaline motives the coronary heart to overcome faster, will boom respiration to deliver more oxygen to the muscle mass, and motives the pores and pores and skin's blood vessels to narrow to save you bleeding. It additionally will increase muscle anxiety and reasons the mouth to dry up. Meanwhile, cortisol allows the body keep energy stages and keeps the man or woman alert.

However, extended exposure to cortisol can damage the mind and the body. High cortisol levels can result in a decrease in dopamine, which can purpose horrible feelings. Therefore, managing the frame's reaction to stress and anxiety is important to avoid long-time period damage.

Cortisol can also have an impact on different elements of the body except the mind. It can lower contamination, that's a tremendous component within the brief time period even as your frame desires to attention on managing a threat. But if cortisol tiers stay excessive for a long time, it is able to purpose a weakened immune device and advanced chance of infections.

High cortisol stages also can have an impact on sleep patterns, main to problem falling or staying asleep. This can further make a contribution to a cycle of strain and terrible health.

In addition, cortisol could have an impact at the reproductive machine, main to reduced libido and disrupted menstrual cycles. It can also affect the increase and repair of bones, major to osteoporosis.

While cortisol may be beneficial inside the short term, persistent pressure and excessive cortisol degrees can negatively impact many factors of fitness. It's crucial to locate strategies to manipulate stress and preserve a healthy way of existence to keep away from the ones horrible results.

The long-time period effects of strain on the thoughts can also purpose changes in behavior. People experiencing chronic stress may additionally moreover additionally end up greater irritable, stressful, or depressed, and they may have hassle napping or experience fatigue. Chronic stress can also result in adjustments in urge for meals, causing some human beings to overeat or lose their urge for food altogether.

In addition to the ones behavioral modifications, chronic stress can bodily have an impact on the body. For instance, it can growth the threat of coronary coronary

coronary heart sickness, stroke, and other persistent health conditions. Stress can also weaken the immune tool, making it less difficult for human beings to get sick.

Overall, even as the stress response may be useful in the short term, continual strain can significantly impact physical and mental fitness. Finding healthy techniques to manipulate pressure, together with exercise, relaxation techniques, and social help, is essential to prevent prolonged-term harm to the body and mind.

LeDoux has moreover positioned every other manner to deal with false alarms. By "extinction education," you could educate the amygdala that the cue it responds to is no longer a threat. Extinction training includes exposing your self to the stimulus that triggers your fear response however in a safe and managed environment. Repeated publicity to the stimulus with none awful results will finally lessen the amygdala's response.

Extinction schooling may be beneficial for treating anxiety problems which incorporates PTSD and phobias. However, it is not a one-size-suits-all solution, and it is able to be hard to apply in positive situations. Other remedies, together with cognitive-behavioral treatment and medicine, may also be necessary.

It's critical to word that strain and tension are ordinary components of existence, and now not all strain is terrible. Stress can negatively have an effect on the mind and frame while it becomes persistent and overwhelming. Taking steps to govern stress, collectively with exercising, mindfulness, and social help, can assist prevent the lengthy-term consequences of pressure at the thoughts.

Interestingly, some other a part of the amygdala, the basal nucleus stria terminalis (BNST), can bypass the important nucleus and keep away from wrongly linking non-threatening stimuli with actual threats. You can activate the BNST and prevent the fight-

or-flight reaction with the useful resource of taking movement. This movement additionally wakes up the left frontal lobe, it's miles more movement-oriented and makes it less tough to experience precise, in assessment to the withdrawal-orientated proper frontal lobe, which makes it much less hard to feel bad. People with anxiety problems will be predisposed to have an excessive amount of interest in the right frontal lobe, that may cause them to enjoy beaten.

To prevent fake alarms and flip off the HPA axis, which controls the frame's stress response, the left prefrontal cortex (PFC) and hippocampus paintings collectively to calm the amygdala. When the proper frontal lobe is too reactive, taking movement and doing a little component beneficial can assist lessen feeling beaten. Ultimately, you can save you the combat-or-flight response and manipulate your emotions through way of acting and activating the BNST and left frontal lobe.

Finding Calm in The Chaos

Although small in share to the relaxation of the body, the brain calls for high-quality power to operate efficiently. It payments for approximately 20% of the body's energy consumption however comprising excellent 3% of its weight. Unfortunately, the thoughts can't keep gas, and therefore, it ought to continuously generate energy as needed. However, the brain can remarkably maximize the usage of available belongings, allowing it to feature effectively even beneath traumatic occasions.

During intervals of immoderate strain, the brain's attentional recognition can also shift from focused processing to prioritizing the perceived danger. In such instances, the mind's number one aim is to extend a way to triumph over worrying situations. This cognitive response can be so severe that human beings won't contemplate the larger photograph of lifestyles. Furthermore, this shift in focus can also result in hasty and impulsive preference-making, in all likelihood essential to destructive consequences.

Excessive tension may be overwhelming, and in hard situations, together with a panic attack, people can also apprehend themselves as having a systematic emergency, including a coronary coronary coronary heart assault. However, it's far critical to have a look at that pressure is a everyday and inevitable a part of lifestyles and isn't typically terrible. Stress may be a beneficial tool to help human beings accomplish their desires, as it motivates them to do so. By fending off stress altogether, one can also become hypersensitive to minor stressors, resulting in undue anxiety. In evaluation, some stress diploma is important to hold productiveness, which includes meeting closing dates and adhering to web site site visitors guidelines. Thus, managing pressure and harnessing its potential can be beneficial for accomplishing personal and professional increase.

Jane determined that mild pressure may be useful and that it could be managed. Stress is vital for the mind to maintain in thoughts essential sports and conditions, however it's far essential to govern it. A mild quantity of stress can help with reminiscence and hobby, on the identical time as an excessive amount of stress can hinder awareness and studying.

Jane found to use a controlled strain stage to enhance her cognitive function. Despite fearing public talking, Jane realized that retaining off it simplest made her more annoying. She commenced to regulate her thinking and use her anxiety to inspire her to stand her fears.

Neuroscience research has set up that an remarkable quantity of hysteria blessings neuroplasticity. Too plenty or too little worry is not beneficial. Instead of warding off anxiety, people should confront it and discover ways to apply it to their gain.

One analogy to bear in thoughts is skiing. You are likelier to fall if you lean too far back for your skis. However, if you lean slightly beforehand, you can manipulate your skis better, even on a steep slope. Similarly, thru using a mild stress degree, people can preserve control of their cognitive functioning, although confronted with difficult events.

Moderate levels of strain can be useful for reminiscence and interest, as studies has tested that the mind dreams some strain to don't forget critical activities and situations. It's essential to manipulate the pressure you enjoy, as too much or too little need to have destructive results.

Utilizing a controlled degree of pressure can decorate cognitive feature. It's commonplace for people to keep away from situations that cause anxiety or pressure, however this behavior can often worsen tension. Instead, humans can exchange their technique and use tension as a motivator to stand their fears and push themselves out of doors their comfort region.

Neuroscientific research indicates that mild anxiety ranges are maximum excessive first-class for neuroplasticity, due to this that too much or too little anxiety is not beneficial for cognitive functioning. An analogy to preserve in thoughts is snowboarding leaning too far again on skis can bring about falls, however leaning slightly forward can beautify manage, even on steep slopes. Similarly, mild strain can help people keep manipulate of their cognitive functioning even in difficult circumstances.

Balancing being too complacent and annoying is critical whilst getting equipped for an exam. A lack of training due to boredom or laziness can purpose horrible performance, at the same time as immoderate fear can prevent gaining knowledge of and retention. This maximum top notch balance is referred to as the "inverted U" or "Yerkes-Dobson curve" in medical phrases.

The inverted U indicates moderate strain and anxiety degrees can gain cognitive function.

This is due to the fact even as the thoughts recollections moderate activation, it produces the right neurochemistry to inspire neuroplasticity and neurogenesis, considering the boom and improvement of the mind.

Rather than warding off pressure and tension, human beings should learn how to control it. When the mind memories mild strain, the neurotransmitters cortisol, CRF, and norepinephrine bind to cellular receptors and boom the hobby of the excitatory neurotransmitter glutamate. This advanced interest inside the hippocampus lets in the float of records and the dynamics at the synapses which are crucial for neuroplasticity.

The more often a message is transmitted alongside the identical pathway, the lots much less hard it turns into for the equal symptoms to fireside and use a good buy plenty much less glutamate. This promotes the wiring collectively of cells and strengthens neural pathways. By learning a manner to manipulate strain and anxiety, humans can promote the boom and health in their brains, major to expanded neuroplasticity and cognitive feature.

Unlocking the Power of Your Parasympathetic Nervous System

The autonomic irritating system is composed of the sympathetic and parasympathetic demanding systems. The former induces satisfaction, even as the latter promotes relaxation. The sympathetic fearful tool triggers the HPA axis and the fight-or-flight reaction at some stage in exceedingly stressful situations. However, this reaction is counterbalanced via what Harvard professor Herbert Benson known as the "rest reaction," that could be a manifestation of the parasympathetic anxious system. This reaction aids in reducing coronary coronary coronary heart, metabolic, and respiratory prices, allowing the frame to lighten up.

When the combat-or-flight response is activated, the body's physiological features, collectively with coronary coronary heart charge, blood stress, metabolism, muscle anxiety, breathing price, and intellectual arousal, all increase. Conversely, at some diploma within the relaxation response, those features lower. The movement precept mentioned in advance activates the BNST and the left PFC, facilitating the parasympathetic anxious machine's ability to calm the body down.

However, human beings with PTSD may additionally additionally enjoy problem transitioning from the sympathetic fearful device to the parasympathetic tool, which can be attributed to the involvement of the PFC and hippocampus. Furthermore, the amygdala may moreover furthermore emerge as more sensitive to annoying conditions due to the annoying revel in.

Breathing in specific techniques can elicit extraordinary emotions. For instance, when feeling stressful, the breathing rate will increase, ensuing in tightness of stomach muscle businesses and decreased chest growth. In my anxiety class, I frequently study human beings who have a bent to speak rapidly with out taking enough time to breathe. As they proceed from one notion to the following, their anxiety tiers spike, which turns on the same neural networks that stimulate anxiety-related thoughts, recollections, and responses. As they speak new subjects, this cycle can reason even greater concerns and fears.

Normally, people take about nine to sixteen breaths in keeping with minute at the same time as resting. However, throughout a panic assault, the respiration rate can growth up to 20-seven breaths in line with minute, fundamental to sensations of numbness, tingling, dry mouth, and lightheadedness. As the breathing and circulatory systems are part of the cardiovascular machine, short respiration can boost up coronary coronary heart fee and heighten tension. Conversely, slowing down respiratory can reduce coronary coronary heart charge, inducing a experience of calmness.

Changing extremely good behavior, which encompass the way you breathe, is crucial to discover ways to lighten up. Shortness of breath is a not unusual symptom of panic, so gaining knowledge of a way to respire in another way is critical. When you breathe too rapid or hyperventilate, your mind and body go through adjustments that could get worse anxiety.

Hyperventilation results in excessive oxygen consumption, reducing carbon dioxide ranges within the blood. Carbon dioxide plays a important feature in preserving the pH degree of your blood. A decrease in pH degree can cause nerve cells to come to be overexcited, main to tension or maybe panic assaults in case you experience that the sensations are from your manage.

Hypocapnic alkalosis is a circumstance because of immoderate lack of carbon dioxide, that could make the blood more alkaline and less acidic. This can purpose decreased blood go along with the flow to tissues due to narrowed blood vessels and reduced oxygen levels, regardless of taking in too much oxygen. Hypocapnic alkalosis can purpose dizziness, lightheadedness, decreased blood go along with the float to the mind, and tingling within the extremities. If panic attacks stand up frequently, the bodily sensations can purpose faster breathing and exacerbate the signs.

Unraveling the Enigma

When you keep away from topics that make you worried, your worry grows over time. This may not make revel in inside the starting, as keeping off the detail for a quick time can lower your tension. However, maintaining off the hassle for a prolonged length permits tension to fester. For instance, your tension might also additionally moreover rapid decrease if you're frightened of assembly new humans and skipping a dinner party. But your worry of assembly strangers can also need to get worse if you maintain to avoid social conditions. Although avoidance may additionally furthermore make you revel in better inside the short time period, it's miles crucial to confront your fears. This is wherein the anomaly is available in. The option to this paradox is exposure, which involves frequently exposing yourself to situations that make you disturbing. By facing your fears, you could become extra acquainted with them, and in the long run, your anxiety will subside.

A similar instance is a battle veteran with PTSD. Avoiding conditions that trigger their anxiety regularly results in a worsening in their symptoms. However, with the useful resource of step by step exposing themselves to the matters that reason them to stressful, they're capable of discover ways to cope. For example, taking note of fireworks may moreover to start with trigger their PTSD symptoms, however with repeated publicity, they're capable of discover ways to partner the sound with excellent tales in desire to trauma. Avoidance and other protection behaviors can get worse anxiety, so it's far essential to confront your fears in choice to run from them.

When you are in a traumatic position, your instinct can be to find a way out of it as short as possible. To avoid similarly tension, you do away with your self from the situation. Assume, for example, which you are in a crowded place and all at once revel in a hurry of tension.

If you feel afraid, leaving the room is an break out addiction you could do. However, your worry will growth as time passes because of the truth you, too, can't cope.

Let's say you're afraid of tension and choose to keep away from it in vicinity of discover ways to cope. As a end result, you can start to word even the smallest symptoms and signs and symptoms of unease and react strongly to them. Because of this, it is frequently known as an tension-willing character trait.

When you have interaction in avoidant behavior, you shy away from situations that could purpose annoying feelings. Suppose, as an example, that your friend has endorsed which you all get together at the residence of one of her distinct buddies. You apprehend that touring your exceptional friend's place will motive you unnecessary tension, so you pass it. That's a method to live smooth of a trouble. Your prolonged-term anxiety will increase as a give up give up end result, as you could in no way examine that the property you worry aren't so horrible if you avoid them.

Procrastination consists of eliminating performing some element because of the truth you preserve in thoughts (incorrectly) that placing it off will lessen your strain tiers. A proper example will be in case you envisage to appearance a friend however waited until the final minute. The more you put topics off till the final minute, the greater worrying you becomes. Since you have been worrying and on element while you in the long run arrived, you may in all likelihood have glad yourself that ready till the remaining minute come to be a smart idea. Isolating your self from the source of your anxiety great heightens your distress.

"Safety behavior" refers to retaining oneself busy or transporting items that make one experience extra consistent. Imagine feeling worrying at a friend's residence after visiting them. You start fiddling collectively together with your headscarf to take your thoughts off topics, hoping to relieve a number of your tension. Taking such precautions is wise. While running in the direction of protection behavior permit you to live in a unmarried region in preference to fleeing, it additionally has the capability to come to be an annoying dependancy. By wearing out this behavior, you are telling your self which you can't manipulate something is making you worrying.

The trouble with searching for to keep away from tension triggers is that doing so prevents you from becoming privy to them. Avoidance of fear is counterproductive in case you want to overcome it.

Avoidance is a sturdy brief-term reinforcer because it reduces anxiety inside the suggest time. This makes it tough to refuse. More strive placed into keeping off what motives tension handiest results in greater convoluted techniques for doing so. The development of agoraphobia, the priority of leaving one's domestic, is a possible impact of excessive avoidance. It's not smooth to break the dependancy of retaining off some element while you start.

Given the ones elements, fending off avoidance may be difficult.

Because avoidance develops right into a dependancy, the extra you have interaction in it, the extra tough it will be to prevent doing so in the future.

At first, appearance, keeping off some detail that causes anxiety appears rational.

Many humans take specific care of you because of the truth they enjoy horrible for you.

Avoiding it, no matter the fact that, only makes the "worry circuit" to your brain extra active. An amygdala arousal due to the concern circuit will growth worry degrees. The OFC investigates the motives of tension to look if amygdala hyperactivity is responsible. The worst form of worry cycle is expert with the aid of humans with OCD, an infection in which traumatic will become obsessive.

Another common approach for managing fear is to try to suppress it. The desire to govern the whole lot would possibly motive avoidance. Anxiety can be avoided high-quality in case you do now not located yourself in a situation in which you are always looking to foresee the destiny. That's wherein topics can get complex in conjunction with your method to save you them. Considering the worst-case conditions, you may revel in anxiety you have not expert earlier than.

The similarly you attempt to interrupt out, the extra you can need to get away. Initially, you simplest reveal your self to analyzing fabric you understand will reason you tension. However, you could quick be exposed to studying material that might purpose distress. Avoiding activities and hobbies will motive your tension is your skip-to approach. You discover ways to avoid conditions that became as soon as cushty after experiencing even a fraction of fear there. Not as masses may be inner your talents for plenty longer. As your circle of have an effect on decreases, your publicity to the matters that strain you outgrow. What in case you push it too far and grow to be with agoraphobia? If it takes area, you'll be too scared to go away the residence.

In a nutshell, spreading fear thru a loss of interest due to heading off triggers surely makes topics worse. The more you keep away from conditions, the more your tension grows, and the extra you avoid conditions, and so forth. It's getting worse as time is going on.

Disrupting this revolving door of bad feelings is the simplest way to advantage mastery over your amygdala. The first step is to confront your anxieties head-on. Keep your alternatives open for coping with subjects that worry you. You'll deliver your self a preventing possibility to conform well to new circumstances.

You can overcome your fear of a few factor by using the usage of managing it head-on yet again.

The fear circuit relaxes even as you endure in thoughts your issues without turning into consumed, and this conduct has been linked to OCD. If you are a worrier, analyzing can help you break out the intricacies of your issues and right into a worldwide of its non-public.

Unlocking Your Frontal Lobe's Power for Positive Change

The mind is a very complex organ comprising severa systems that artwork collectively to control our thoughts, emotions, and behaviors. One of the most critical structures is the prefrontal cortex (PFC), responsible for selection-making, attention, and emotional law. The PFC works with the hippocampus, which permits us shape and keep memories, to provide situational that means to our experiences.

For instance, while we come upon a possibly threatening situation, collectively with seeing a figure inside the dark, our sympathetic anxious device kicks in, and our combat-or-flight response is delivered on. The PFC then analyzes the scenario and makes a preference whether the decide is a chance. The hippocampus allows us recollect the context of the scenario, which consist of the decide's vicinity and surrounding devices. If the determine seems harmless, the PFC signs the amygdala to lighten up, and the strain response is have become off.

How we speak approximately our studies will have an impact on how our thoughts abilities. When we time and again inform ourselves horrible reminiscences, together with "This is tough," "I can not do it," or "This will go incorrect," our brains start to red meat up those neural circuits, making them more potent. This terrible self-communicate can emerge as automated and ingrained, affecting our fashionable highbrow health and nicely-being.

Our stories consist of 3 thoughts: automatic thoughts, assumptions, and center ideals. Automatic thoughts are like quick tapes that run through our minds, regularly with out us being conscious. They can be outstanding or lousy and can have an impact on our mood and conduct. Assumptions are ideals that bridge the distance between our automated mind and middle ideals. They are not as deep-rooted as center ideals however notwithstanding the reality which have an effect on how we see ourselves and the arena spherical us.

Core ideals are our most deeply held beliefs about ourselves and the arena. They can be top notch or bad, shaping how we assume, experience, and behave. Negative middle ideals, which include "I'm no longer suitable sufficient," "I'm unlovable," or "I'm a failure," may be associated with anxiety and melancholy. These ideals may be tough to change, but with practice and staying strength, it's far feasible to rewire the thoughts and boom more exceptional center beliefs.

Cognitive-behavioral remedy (CBT) is a shape of remedy that specializes in converting horrible idea styles and ideals. It dreams to assist people turn out to be aware about their automatic thoughts, challenge their assumptions, and reframe their center beliefs extra genuinely. CBT can correctly address anxiety, despair, and one-of-a-kind highbrow fitness conditions.

The way we speak approximately our evaluations may have a profound effect on our intellectual health and properly-being. By changing our automatic mind and assumptions and reframing our middle beliefs, we are able to rewire our brains and increase a powerful outlook on lifestyles. CBT is a effective tool to help people conquer awful belief patterns and lead happier, greater pleasurable lives.

Chapter 6: Embrace The Grind

"Neurons that hearth collectively, twine collectively. By taking within the specific, we will use our minds to alternate our brains in procedures which will assist us be happier and additional effective."

Dr. Rick Hanson

Our emotions significantly have an effect on how we understand, anticipate, and recollect topics. When we experience a specific feeling, the neurons chargeable for that emotion start to fireplace collectively, connecting with other neurons accountable for mind and recollections. This creates a neural network, which may be seen as an attractor that attracts in our thoughts, emotions, and recollections and affects our behavior. The more potent this neural network will become, the more likely we are able to keep feeling the identical way.

However, it's miles vital to be aware that this neural community can also worsen and end up extra difficult to break out of if we do no longer stop it. For example, you're going for walks past due for a own family dinner you are no longer captivated with attending. While driving in rush-hour visitors, you comprehend your fuel tank is kind of empty, which adds to your strain and anger. You pull proper right into a gas station great to look a protracted line of cars geared up to top off. Some human beings take their time, making you even more pissed off and worrying.

As you continue to think about your scenario, your feelings end up more immoderate, and you revel in worse. You begin to fear about your aunt's reaction for your cast off and sense unhappy while you do not forget how upset she'll be. These horrible feelings pork up the neural network keeping you in a terrible mood.

However, a danger come upon with a lady at the gas station helps you escape it. At first, you are irritated together along with her for leaving her car at the pump to run into the shop. But even as you have a look at that her toddler has no hair, you understand he must undergo chemotherapy for maximum cancers. Suddenly, your thoughts-set shifts, and you feel empathy for the lady and her toddler. When you come, you rush into the store to shop for the boy a drink and deliver it to him. He gives you a unhappy smile, however you enjoy accurate about yourself for assisting out.

This story illustrates how clean it's far to fall proper into a horrible emotional united states of america and the manner challenging it could be to break out it. The greater we take satisfaction in terrible emotions, the more potent the neural network that allows them turns into. These emotions can last for hours, days, weeks, or possibly months, foremost to the negativity that permeates our thoughts, reminiscences, and moves.

If we usually generally tend to experience a selected emotion maximum of the time, it will become the inspiration of our lives, the middle round which our mind and movements revolve. For example, if we've had been given been feeling sad for an extended duration, it becomes our default mood, shaping how we perceive the vicinity and influencing our conduct.

However, finding a balance among acknowledging our feelings and transferring on with our lives is important. For example, if we've got lost a person near us, feeling unhappy is everyday and natural. Still, we should locate strategies to cope and skip beforehand without getting caught in a horrible emotional united states.

One manner to break out of terrible emotional states is to "go together with the waft the needle" via changing the neural network that lets in them. There are severa methods to do that, together with priming high-quality moods, using moderate treatment, building narratives, taking motion, workout, wiring powerful questioning, and attractive in social sports.

Priming top notch moods is a manner of starting your day well. You can start your day with powerful affirmations or meditations that assist you location a nice tone for the relaxation of the day. This exercise will now not simplest help you experience better about your self, however it will additionally assist you make bigger a more first rate outlook on lifestyles.

Light chemistry is the test of the way light impacts our moods and conduct. Exposure to daytime or brilliant mild can enhance our temper and strength ranges. This is because of the reality daytime triggers the producing of serotonin, a neurotransmitter that regulates mood, sleep, and urge for food.

Constructing narratives is a manner of reframing bad events in a extra superb mild. This cognitive-behavioral method involves identifying terrible perception patterns and changing them with greater wonderful ones.

Taking action is a way of breaking out bad idea styles thru performing some factor powerful. This may be as clean as strolling or calling a chum. By taking movement, you're interrupting the bad cycle of mind and changing them with more outstanding ones.

Aerobic boosting consists of getting your coronary heart price up through exercise. This may be anything from going for a jog to taking a dance elegance. Aerobic exercise has been proven to enhance temper and decrease signs and symptoms and symptoms of melancholy and tension.

Wiring high-quality thinking includes deliberately specializing in splendid thoughts and feelings, which might be as clean as repeating high-quality affirmations to yourself or specializing in glad reminiscences. By wiring excessive outstanding wondering, you strengthen the neural pathways helping exceptional feelings.

Social treatment includes the electricity of social guide to decorate our temper and brand new nicely-being. This might be as easy as spending time with buddies or turning into a member of a resource organization. By connecting with others, we are able to percentage our struggles and find out comfort in knowing we aren't on my own.

Unlocking the Power of Priming Positive Moods

Changing your brain's capability may be finished with the aid of stimulating high high-quality emotions and behaving luckily, even even as you do no longer revel in find it irresistible. If you're feeling low and preserving off social conditions, spending time with buddies can enhance your mood. Smiling can spark off additives of your thoughts that deal with glad feelings. Researcher Kelly Lambert has highlighted the importance of the strive-pushed reward circuit inside the thoughts in combatting depression. This circuit contains the nucleus accumbens, striatum, and prefrontal cortex (PFC). The nucleus accumbens enables with emotions and memories and performs a function in behaviors which might be tough to stop, while the striatum is worried in movement and is a link amongst our emotions and movements. The PFC is accountable for fixing troubles and making plans and alternatives.

The strive-pushed praise circuit links conduct with rewards, and turning off the accumbens can purpose a loss of delight. Similarly, moving slowly turns off the striatum, and a loss of reputation turns off the PFC. Cognitive-behavioral therapists have extended suggested depressed people to be extra active, which has been determined to reduce melancholy. This is referred to as "behavioral activation" and appears to spark off the attempt-driven rewards circuit related to the accumbens, striatum, and PFC.

Studies have decided a link among the asymmetry of the 2 factors of the mind and melancholy. Neurology has validated that a stroke on the left factor of the brain may be devastating and reason depression, on the same time as a stroke on the proper thing is a whole lot much less intense and motives less depression. The left PFC is accountable for nicely emotions and actions, at the identical time due to the fact the proper PFC is associated with horrible emotions and state of no activity. Depression is related to a slowing down of the left PFC and an boom inside the tempo of the proper PFC.

The mind's left hemisphere is answerable for language, excellent emotions, and making enjoy of what is going on. In assessment, the proper hemisphere thinks approximately the whole international, that could reason negative wondering. Behavioral activation regarding the left PFC is a key way to cope with depression.

Putting yourself available and seeking out to be glad can assist combat despair. Neural pathways connect facial muscle tissue, cranial nerves, subcortical regions, and the cortex. Tightening the muscle groups at the right aspect of the face can spark off the left hemisphere, this is much more likely to make you enjoy glad. On the other hand, tightening the muscle mass at the left issue of the face can activate the proper hemisphere, leading to lousy thinking.

Activating the strive-pushed reward circuit within the thoughts with the useful resource of behaving thankfully and being extra active can assist fight melancholy. It is critical to area your self on hand, no matter the fact that it way "setting on a glad face." The left PFC is liable for first rate emotions and taking motion, making behavioral activation a key way to address melancholy.

Contralateral Functions

The idea of contralateral functioning describes the connection some of the facial muscle tissues on one trouble of the face and the opportunity hemisphere of the mind. This technique the right facial muscle mass are associated with the left hemisphere, while the left facial muscle agencies are related to the right hemisphere. This concept is exemplified with the useful resource of the Mona Lisa's enigmatic smile, in which the proper side of her face appears happy on the identical time as the left aspect seems sad or impartial. By turning into a member of the two halves of her face, the difference many of the elements will become more apparent.

Research shows that the mind's left hemisphere is greater worried in processing great emotions, whilst the proper hemisphere is associated with poor feelings. Therefore, every side of the face can show one-of-a-kind emotions counting on the more energetic hemisphere. Studies have validated that even if you pressure your self to grin or frown, it is able to have an impact on your emotions. This is because of the truth facial expressions can ship alerts to the mind that set off the corresponding subcortical and cortical regions, major to a change in temper. Thus, setting on a grin can truely make you revel in better.

Moreover, the thoughts's left hemisphere is likewise associated with movement, at the same time as the right hemisphere is greater passive. Taking movement can help humans experience a whole lot much less unhappy, at the same time as being passive can result in emotions of sadness. For example, at the same time as a person is depressed, their left frontal lobe, accountable for selection-making and movement, won't function as well because it want to. Therefore, wearing out incredible sports activities that stimulate the left frontal lobe can assist damage the cycle of unhappiness and sell a extra remarkable outlook on existence.

Interestingly, the left location of imaginative and prescient is related to the proper hemisphere, even as the right situation is associated with the left hemisphere. Therefore, on the identical time as you look to the left, your right hemisphere is activated, and at the same time as you appearance to the proper, your left hemisphere is activated. This connection a few of the sector of vision and mind hemisphere activation can impact how we understand and process emotions.

Finally, humor can be a effective device in changing our temper and attitude. Research has confirmed that humor can help us detach from negative mind and feelings, permitting us to approach situations more lightheartedly. Reading comedic cloth or searching funny movies can efficaciously shift our mood from disappointment to happiness. However, it's far crucial to be aware that humor should never be used to belittle or harm others.

Exploring the Hilarious Side of Science

Laughter has a effective impact in your biochemistry and has been determined to decrease the quantity of cortisol, the strain hormone, to your body. Additionally, laughter can boom the levels of immunoglobulin, natural killer (NK) cells, and plasma cytokine gamma interferon. Immunoglobulin is an important part of your immune gadget that enables to combat off infections, and NK cells pick out and kill unusual cells inside the immunosurveillance manner. Finally, plasma cytokine gamma interferon allows to coordinate and manage anti-mobile sports activities activities and activates specific factors of the immune gadget.

Furthermore, mastering to snicker at your self can decorate your self-photograph and decrease your stress. When you do not take yourself too seriously, it allows you to look yourself inside the context of a bigger picture. You can also permit flow of youngster troubles and keep away from sweating the small stuff. You can sense higher and extra amazing thru growing a humorousness. Spending as loads time as feasible in a effective and first-rate state of mind is critical to make it much less complicated as a manner to keep that mind-set. Encouraging exceptional thoughts, attitudes, and movements that result in an high-quality mood will can help you to preserve a top notch outlook.

Exploring the Powerful Impact of Light on Positive Mood

Depression is a common intellectual health condition that influences many human beings. Unfortunately, human beings with depression often isolate themselves from the outdoor international through very last curtains, warding off daytime, and staying indoors. However, depriving oneself of natural moderate may additionally moreover get worse melancholy symptoms and symptoms.

The retina behind the eye is important in informing the mind of the mild situations outside. This facts is then transmitted to the pineal gland, which releases melatonin to assist modify sleep patterns. In terrific mild conditions, the pineal gland does no longer release melatonin, growing serotonin degrees, it's miles crucial for keeping particular intellectual health.

Research has confirmed that depression is attached to low serotonin ranges. Seasonal affective infection (SAD) is a type of despair that takes region in the path of wintry climate because of low mild conditions. People with

SAD often experience greater depressed, that's greater commonplace in regions with fewer sunlight hours within the course of iciness.

To beautify one's highbrow fitness, spending greater time inside the solar is crucial, as natural slight is useful to the mind's chemistry. Sitting below a entire-spectrum light is an powerful remedy alternative for people with SAD. While daylight hours is the excellent possibility, human beings living in areas with a whole lot much less light ultimately of wintry climate may also moreover need to undergo in thoughts a complete-spectrum mild to assist fight SAD.

Getting sufficient nutrients D is crucial for the immune system and large properly-being. Sunlight is an amazing supply of nutrition D, and people who spend extra time outside in herbal light can decorate their popular health. Therefore, human beings want to try and get as lots natural moderate as viable in the course of the day, even definitely thru starting the curtains or taking a quick stroll outside.

The Transformative Effects of Exercise on Mood

Regular exercising gives numerous bodily and intellectual advantages. Exercise enhances blood motion through growing the quantity of oxygen the blood consists of, resulting in superior intellectual readability and decreased strain levels. Additionally, exercise must make the frame loads less acidic, in order to increase energy ranges.

Stretching and exercise moreover beautify blood waft to the muscle groups. Stretching forces the oxygen-horrific blood to return to the lungs to be re-oxygenated. This manner advantages the muscle groups via using way of providing them with freshly oxygenated blood, reducing muscle anxiety, and improving their typical health.

Physical workout triggers the manufacturing of norepinephrine, a hormone an amazing manner to increase coronary heart price, which helps to raise the mood. People who be anxious thru melancholy and anxiety often benefit from workout, as it is able to assist to alleviate signs.

Numerous research have validated that exercise definitely affects the brain's cognitive capabilities, collectively with neurogenesis and neuroplasticity. These benefits may also have an enduring impact at the brain and enhance extensive cognitive function.

Physical interest does no longer ought to be restrained to structured workout workouts. Walking unexpectedly, taking the stairs, and doing circle of relatives chores can all be effective kinds of exercising. It is essential to consider that everyday workout and a exquisite outlook ought to make a giant distinction in a single's normal well-being.

The Effects of Constructing Narratives

The brain has outstanding aspects that perform top notch abilities. The right facet is liable for feelings and taking in facts holistically, at the identical time because the left translates studies and makes use of language to talk. Psychologists name this system storytelling, in which we label and provide which means that to life events. By telling exquisite reminiscences, we're capable of rewire our brains to attention at the excessive top notch elements of our studies.

Our left hemisphere controls language and locations our reminiscences into phrases. By framing our research certainly, we're able to set off the left hemisphere's wonderful bias and promote awesome questioning. Every time we don't forget some thing, we trade it, and the left hemisphere is chargeable for assisting us create a amazing narrative approximately what we need to recollect.

Both aspects of the thoughts are essential and must paintings together like equals. The proper hemisphere is crucial for emotional reports and remembering our enjoy of self. Still, it wishes the left hemisphere's attention to element and first rate spin to help us in reality reframe our reviews.

The Potential of Your Beliefs

Beliefs and belief strategies can drastically impact one's emotional well-being, and research have showed that changing one's mind can result in modifications in how one feels. Research using brain imaging has located that severa treatments for depression have exceptional outcomes on thoughts interest. For instance, cognitive-behavioral remedy (CBT) has been verified to increase hippocampus interest even as lowering hobby inside the overactive OFC. By changing horrible mind with extra realistic ones, CBT facilitates to keep new, high-quality, and sensible thoughts inside the hippocampus, at the same time as antidepressant treatment won't have the identical impact.

Although antidepressants can be powerful for some people, they regularly require lengthy-time period use, and lots of people do not revel in any improvement in their signs and signs. The placebo effect, in which a person's notion in treatment can produce outstanding consequences, has been drastically studied in medicine. Placebos produce among sixty 5 and eighty% of the consequences of antidepressants. The energy of notion is specially effective in treating highbrow fitness situations, because of the fact the placebo impact is highbrow.

In a have a have a take a look at completed via researchers at the University of Toronto, depressed individuals who believed they have been taking a powerful antidepressant but were taking a placebo nonetheless expert changes in their symptoms and symptoms and symptoms and signs related to modifications in mind activity. The placebo effect demonstrates the massive effect of ideals on one's opinions, every mentally and physical.

Overall, converting one's thoughts and ideals can result in great improvements in emotional nicely-being. While antidepressants can be useful for some human beings, the strength of notion established with the aid of the placebo impact shows that the impact of idea strategies on intellectual health isn't always to be underestimated.

Sparking Joy: The Power of Wiring Positive Thinking in Your Mind

Our thoughts and feelings are inextricably associated, and horrible mind can bring about terrible feelings, whilst incredible thoughts can result in powerful emotions. This connection is the muse of Cognitive Behavioral Therapy (CBT), a remedy modality that targets to accurate terrible idea patterns and decorate emotional properly-being.

CBT is a nicely-mounted, evidence-primarily based approach to treating despair, anxiety, and specific intellectual health situations. CBT goals to assist individuals emerge as aware of and project bad idea patterns, converting them with extra excellent and practical ones. By changing how we think, we are capable of change how we experience.

One of the vital component components of CBT is cognitive restructuring. This includes figuring out bad thoughts and beliefs and changing them with more extremely good and realistic ones. For example, assume someone believes they will be nugatory because they made a mistake at artwork. In that case, a therapist may venture this notion with the resource of way of asking the person to hold in thoughts whether or not they might say the identical element to a chum who made a similar mistake. This permits to reframe the horrible perception in a more extremely good slight.

There are severa common cognitive distortions that human beings with despair and tension frequently revel in. These embody polarized thinking (seeing matters as all actual or all terrible), overgeneralization (drawing massive conclusions primarily based on restricted evidence), personalization (attributing terrible activities to oneself), and catastrophizing (assuming the worst possible final results). By figuring out and hard those cognitive distortions, individuals can enhance their mood and decrease signs and symptoms and signs and symptoms of depression and tension.

Another essential issue of CBT is behavioral activation. This consists of growing engagement in quality sports activities like exercise, socializing, and interests. By developing superb reviews, people can enhance their temper and reduce terrible questioning patterns.

In addition to cognitive restructuring and behavioral activation, several other techniques can assist address melancholy and anxiety. One such approach is mindfulness, which involves listening to the existing 2d without judgment. Mindfulness can assist human beings come to be more privy to their mind and feelings, permitting them to discover terrible belief patterns and replace them with more fantastic ones.

Another technique is trouble-fixing, which includes breaking down problems into viable components and developing techniques to cope with them. This can be particularly useful for human beings beaten through bad conditions or occasions.

Ultimately, CBT targets to assist humans increase a extra pleasant and sensible outlook on lifestyles. By identifying and hard negative concept patterns, task amazing sports activities activities, and gaining expertise of new coping strategies, people can enhance their mood and decrease symptoms of depression and tension. While CBT won't be powerful for absolutely everyone, it's miles a notably recognized and proof-based remedy modality that has helped infinite human beings decorate their highbrow health and nicely-being.

Building Bridges: The Art of Social Connections

As humans, we are social creatures, and the guide of others can undoubtedly effect our properly-being. Empathy is a natural response this is facilitated by way of the usage of replicate neurons. It is not unusual to want to withdraw from social interactions whilst feeling down, but this can bring about an overactive right prefrontal cortex, hindering our capability to attain this. Positive relationships are essential to feeling suitable. From the instant we are born, our brains are careworn to are trying to find out bonding research with others. The orbitofrontal cortex (OFC) is a thoughts region closely concerned in social bonding, and it responds definitely to appropriate relationships at the same time as experiencing withdrawals whilst strained or broken relationships.

Recent studies suggests that the OFC includes herbal opiates that help us enjoy in the direction of others. When we experience appeal or closeness with a person, our brains release dopamine, which makes us enjoy right. The neurohormone oxytocin is likewise activated sooner or later of bodily touch or cuddling, reinforcing the high fine emotions related to social bonding. Thus, suitable relationships are similar to social remedy.

When feeling down, keeping apart ourselves from others may be tempting, but this may be counterproductive. Just as we take medicinal drug at the same time as we're physical sick, attempting to find social useful resource inside the route of difficult times is critical to improve our emotional nicely-being.

Take Action

Recent research has suggested that anger can be a motivating stress that wakes up the thoughts's left frontal lobe, that may motive a more even balance of hobby most of the frontal lobes. This shift can result in a more high pleasant outlook on lifestyles, specially even as people take powerful movement in reaction to their anger.

If a person feels down or unhappy, taking movement may be a effective way to beautify their temper. Individuals can shift from a "can't do some thing" mindset to an "I can" mind-set with the aid of way of doing something inexperienced. In comparison, passivity cannot at once make a contribution to poor emotions and pessimism, despite the fact that someone believes they're defensive power with the useful useful resource of being passive.

To beautify one's mood, it's far useful to recognition on the tremendous temper country one would really like to experience and then take movement to gain it. Moving from a passive to an energetic usa, or from the right frontal lobe to the left frontal lobe, may be tough but profitable. Pushing oneself to have interaction in activities, even though they do no longer experience discover it impossible to resist, can help create excellent momentum.

Creating first rate testimonies, connecting with others, and taking note of incredible studies can all help twine extremely good thoughts into the thoughts. It's important to stay privy to one's mood country and take motion to avoid slipping lower back into awful styles.

Sticking to a cutting-edge plan may be difficult whilst faced with adversity, however keeping wish that the plan will paintings and taking motion can help people climate the storm. Practicing feeding one's mind can little by little create a modern-day default temper america of america that is extra extraordinary and useful. By retaining a pleasing outlook, people can technique demanding situations as opportunities for increase and resilience.

Chapter 7: Memory Mastery

"Memory works a bit bit like a Wikipedia page: you could skip in there and trade it, but so can distinct human beings."

Dr. Elizabeth Loftus

According to a Roper ballot , many people struggle with reminiscence lapses, collectively with stepping into a room and forgetting why they went there. While it is able to look like our recollections are deteriorating, it is vital to take a look at that reminiscence can't be misplaced or positioned, however as an opportunity it may be progressed or allowed to get worse over the years.

In current-day rapid-paced international, with constant distractions from cellular telephones, instantaneous messaging, and media overload, it could be hard to reputation and hold data. It is vital to keep away from getting distracted and live present, centered, and prepared to improve reminiscence. Some powerful methods to enhance reminiscence embody enhancing interest competencies, using special strategies which incorporates mnemonics, and know-how how wonderful types of memory artwork.

On the other hand, numerous topics do no longer artwork concerning reminiscence improvement. Multitasking, as an example, may be damaging to memory as it may motive forgetting critical facts. It is likewise unrealistic to expect memory to improve with none try on our detail, and memory calls for everyday use to stay sturdy. Additionally, memories aren't static and may be altered or misplaced over time if not retrieved or strengthened.

How Attention Serves because the Gateway to Our Memories

Attention is the critical element to unlocking our thoughts's capability to alternate and adapt through neuroplasticity. We can rewire our brains to decorate cognitive feature, enhance reminiscence, and increase new capabilities through paying interest. In evaluation, distractions can impair our hobby and strolling reminiscence, decreasing our capacity to maintain new records and increase new neural connections.

The frontal lobes manual our interest and determine what data have to be saved in memory. The prefrontal cortex (PFC), in particular the Dorsolateral prefrontal cortex (DLPFC), plays a critical position in preserving running reminiscence. Working reminiscence holds quick-time period reminiscences associated with what our minds are running on presently. We use strolling reminiscence to connect our stories and make revel in of them. The DLPFC acts as a command center and determines what information is important to endure in thoughts. It works collectively with the hippocampus to consolidate recollections into prolonged-term memory.

The neurotransmitters norepinephrine and dopamine play a huge function in our potential to pay hobby and bear in mind critical statistics. When we need to bear in mind something, dopamine and norepinephrine help us attention and feel traumatic, main to higher interest and memory retention. These neurotransmitters are launched whilst we encounter a completely unique or emotionally big occasion, making us pay greater hobby to the situation and don't forget it higher. For example, assume we hear that the stock we offered is about to drop soon. In that case, our mind releases dopamine and norepinephrine, making us pay more hobby to the facts and recollect it higher.

In assessment, distractions, inclusive of receiving a textual content message or e-mail notification, can disrupt our going for walks reminiscence and hobby, primary to hassle in consolidating records into lengthy-term memory. Our running reminiscence has a constrained capability, and distractions can fast pinnacle off the strolling reminiscence, leaving little region for logo spanking new facts. Therefore, it is vital to get rid of any distractions which could interfere with our hobby and working memory.

To decorate our memory and sell neuroplasticity, we should pay whole interest to the challenge. The greater important a few factor is to us, the much more likely we are capable of recollect it in the end. If we fail to pay attention, the door to our memory stays closed, and we can not switch facts from brief-time period to prolonged-term memory. Paying interest, we engage our mind's neural circuits and enhance the connections amongst neurons, improving cognitive characteristic and memory retention.

Several elements can impair our attention and working memory, lowering our capability to hold new data and growth new neural connections. Stress, anxiety, and shortage of sleep can impair interest and walking memory, reducing our capability to pay hobby and technique new records. Therefore, it is important to manipulate strain, get sufficient sleep, and have interaction in activities that promote relaxation and mental clarity, which include meditation and yoga.

Furthermore, carrying out sports that sell cognitive stimulation, which encompass studying a present day language, gambling a musical device, or solving puzzles, can decorate hobby and operating reminiscence. These sports mission our mind's neural circuits and promote the development of latest connections, improving cognitive feature and reminiscence retention.

Attention is crucial for promoting neuroplasticity and reminiscence consolidation. Our frontal lobes, in particular the DLPFC, are crucial in guiding our hobby and keeping walking memory. Paying hobby, we have interplay our mind's neural circuits and improve the connections between neurons, improving cognitive characteristic and memory retention. However, distractions, stress, and lack of sleep can impair our interest and on foot reminiscence, lowering our ability to maintain new facts and increase new neural connections. Therefore, coping with pressure, getting enough sleep, and engaging in sports activities sports that promote cognitive stimulation to decorate hobby and jogging memory are critical.

What Are the Types of Memory?

There exist severa variations among strolling memory and lengthy-term memory. The primary assessment lies within the duration of memory storage, and a few different huge version is the garage capability. Working reminiscence has a confined garage area, at the equal time as prolonged-time period memory garage is not a undertaking.

Long-term reminiscence can be likened to a continuously growing library. This is because of the reality long-term memories are not restricted to particular thoughts regions; instead, they seem like fashioned at the same time as multiple thoughts areas are concurrently engaged. As I will difficult, reminiscences regularly adhere to precise mind regions. Thus, whether or now not an experience, a piece of statistics, or an emotional sensation is stored in prolonged-time period memory is based upon on how the diverse neural structures collaborate.

Learning and remembering are carefully related competencies. As relationships with others deepen, shared recollections are expressed and stated. Declarative reminiscence involves recalling beyond occurrences, together with activities, information, imagery, or content. Semantic reminiscence relates to the recollection of language-related items. Episodic memory entails recalling numerous elements of 1's past simultaneously. These specific memories may be outstanding as follows:

• Episodic reminiscence is remembering a paper cut incident.

• Declarative reminiscence is recalling how the paper reduce passed off.

• Semantic reminiscence is remembering the terms used to provide an explanation for the paper reduce to a person.

Emotional memory emerges while sturdy emotions are related to episodic reminiscence. Procedural reminiscence offers with the recollection of frequently performed movements, like the use of a motorbike or writing one's name. These reminiscence subsystems may be labeled as prolonged-time period memory types, however additionally they may be grouped into fantastic classes: express and implicit. Recognizing this distinction is important for enhancing reminiscence skills. Explicit memory encompasses data and expressed studies, at the equal time as implicit reminiscence includes way and emotional memory.

Some implicit reminiscences, together with emotional memories, are fashioned rapidly, like trauma due to an assault. In evaluation, procedural recollections, like gaining knowledge of to play the cello, require massive exercising to make bigger.

The hippocampus typically stores specific recollections and generates new mind based totally mostly on received know-how and information. Without this functionality, every day may be a completely unique enjoy, and though first of all attractive, this will be undesirable. For example, Henry Molaison, one of the most famous patients in neurology and neuropsychology records (known as "HM" within the studies literature), has taught us an lousy lot about the hippocampus and specific memory.

After undergoing mind surgical procedure as a more youthful person, Henry out of place the potential to shape new, outstanding recollections. At age 9, he modified into struck with the resource of a vehicle and eventually skilled uncontrollable seizures. In 1953, in advance than the hippocampus' function become properly-installation, a neurosurgeon eliminated Henry's right and left hippocampus to mitigate the seizures. While the surgical remedy progressed Henry's seizures, he want to now not don't forget humans. If he briefly conversed with a stranger who left the room and lower back, Henry might have no recollection of the stumble upon.

Henry still retained recollections of remote past sports and competencies. For example, he want to navigate his community and bypass decrease back domestic, albeit now not immediately. He might be shown a selected motion and, on the identical time as requested to perform it later, would possibly execute it higher than inside the direction of the initial training. However, he may not keep in thoughts ever attempting it earlier than.

Neuroscience has decided, thru numerous tests completed via manner of neuropsychologist Brenda Milner, that the hippocampus plays a vital function in storing and retrieving memories. The hippocampus is important for forming a shiny memory of a cutting-edge event however isn't required for recalling an older autobiographical reminiscence.

The hippocampus is a essential issue of the growing old gadget. As humans age, the hippocampus shrinks through the years. Many Alzheimer's sufferers lose their declarative recollections, however a few, like Henry, maintain a few procedural memories. They hold to undergo in mind ordinary actions but warfare to undergo in thoughts current existence events. Emotionally large sports are much more likely to be remembered prolonged-term because of the reality they regularly preserve personal relevance and evoke more pride. Moreover, emotional occasions elicit physiological responses, along with advanced blood glucose stages, helping reminiscence consolidation.

Emotional activities make lasting impressions at the mind, changing brain function and facilitating memory retention. To don't forget some thing effectively, an emotional connection is critical. Consequently, emotionally charged activities are more with out troubles remembered due to their in my view massive problem subjects and heightened pleasure.

Fear is often related to the neural networks that keep emotional reminiscences. As cited in Chapter 2, the subcortical pathways connecting the thalamus (the thoughts's important hub) to the amygdala are accountable for classically conditioned fear responses to auditory and seen stimuli. New York University researcher Joseph LeDoux said, "This circuit bypasses the cortex and is, consequently, a subcortical mechanism for emotional mastering."

While the amygdala is crucial for emotional learning, it does no longer play a extraordinary feature in most declarative reminiscence methods. Conversely, the cortex isn't required to growth conditioned worry but is critical for its elimination. In different terms, worry may be discovered unconsciously but not unlearned with out conscious cognizance. Thus, the cortex is vital for regulating the amygdala to overcome anxiety.

Emotional conditioning can yield numerous effects based totally mostly on the person's emotional country on the time. For instance, if norepinephrine ranges are excessive, conditioning occurs extra unexpectedly, and the conditioned response is located quicker and persists longer.

Like considered one of a type animals, humans can have a look at responsibilities that require the amygdala activation however now not the hippocampus. However, they cannot examine obligations that require the amygdala however no longer the hippocampus.

Through its interactions with the HPA axis, the amygdala stimulates present day hobby and mobilizes the entire thoughts-frame gadget. Even if an occasion does no longer elicit an emotional reaction, it is able to although be remembered as an episode. When the mind functions optimally, the amygdala fosters the precise emotional u . S . For reminiscence retention. Experiencing that emotional america of the usa over again will increase the likelihood of recalling express facts associated with that feeling.

Most humans have little to no recollection in their first 3 to 5 years, and Sigmund Freud misidentified this phenomenon as "childish amnesia." However, those memories have now not been forgotten or suppressed; they stay unconscious and most effective resurface at the same time as precipitated with the useful useful resource of emotional responses. Thus, the implicit memory machine develops before the encoding of express recollections.

Many emotional dispositions and belief strategies are rooted in implicit reminiscence. For example, a desire for chickening out in response to the struggle can also additionally evolve with cognitive improvement and revel in. Still, its implicit feature (preserving restricted connections to others) will possibly live unchanged until the social brain tool is intentionally altered through neuroplasticity. As a end result, whilst fear conditioning and procedural analyzing get up concurrently (in all likelihood unbeknownst to the man or woman and earlier than the whole development of episodic studying), teenagers behavior and conditioned responses may be inadvertently obtained.

Many emotional reactions and behavioral patterns taken into consideration inherent persona traits are implicit recollections. As behavior, they will be hard to alternate without huge try, along with using the FEED approach. Insight by myself does not deliver smooth get admission to to implicit memories, nor does it usually regulate them. Unconscious strategies play a vast position in all relationships due to the truth stories and reactions are frequently primarily based on recollections that human beings are unaware they very own.

Procedural memory is apparent even as you possibly can consequences examine a ebook (supplied no particular responsibilities are being finished concurrently). Procedural memory lets in for analyzing an internet page or with out retaining the content material fabric, because it become acquired while first of all suffering with letters and phrases.

Procedural memory is wonderful from declarative and episodic reminiscence in severa crucial strategies. Unlike declarative and episodic reminiscence, which consist of remembering beyond activities or evaluations, procedural reminiscence lets in for the recollection of located abilties, collectively with studying, gargling, typing, the usage of a motorbike, and extra. Procedural learning does now not necessitate know-how of the content fabric; as an opportunity, it focuses on remembering a manner to perform specific obligations. With sufficient workout, procedural memory permits the execution of severa sports sports automatically and with out aware concept.

Procedural learning is likewise important for person development, which includes the brilliant consistency of behavior, feelings, and mind someone well-known through the years.

To make sure that prolonged-time period memory is primarily based mostly on procedural memory, the subsequent 3 steps must be taken:

Encoding a reminiscence: Sometimes known as "coding a memory," this step takes area while analyzing a ultra-present day ability, inclusive of using a motorcycle for the number one time.

Consolidating a memory: At this degree, the obtained knowledge is recorded for destiny use, as inside the case of studying to journey a motorcycle.

Retrieving a memory: The stored memory is probably recalled the following time the understanding is wanted, which incorporates whilst the use of a motorcycle again.

Having extraordinary among implicit and explicit memory, we're capable of now delve deeper into the topic of precise reminiscence.

The Magic of Associations and Mnemonics

The human mind is an top notch organ storing massive amounts of statistics. However, reminiscence is not a static gadget; it's far a dynamic gadget that requires the thoughts to continuously make new connections amongst neurons. This way is known as neuroplasticity. Neuroplasticity is the mind's ability to reorganize itself with the useful resource of forming new neural connections in the route of life. In one in every of a type terms, each time you research a few trouble new or don't forget something, your mind is bodily changing.

Memory is the foundation of analyzing, and the studying way can be futile without the capability to maintain in mind statistics. Luckily, a few strategies can assist enhance reminiscence and decorate keep in mind. These strategies are based totally on the thoughts of neuroplasticity and consist of making new neural connections to resource memory maintain in mind.

One of the thrilling subjects approximately reminiscence is that it is associative. This way that recalling a reminiscence triggers one among a type associated recollections, growing a series of connections. Associations with photos, thoughts, and feelings shape these connections. Improving memory involves growing robust establishments that may be without difficulty recalled.

One technique that is powerful in improving reminiscence don't forget is the usage of mnemonics. Mnemonics are reminiscence aids that use institutions to help maintain in mind data. The exceptional mnemonics are those which can be a laugh and notable. By making records memorable, you can make it less complicated to don't forget. Throughout facts, many mnemonics have been used. Here are 4 which might be clean to preserve in thoughts:

1. Pegs: Pegs are like hooks that join a difficult-to-consider phrase to an less complicated-to-keep in mind phrase. For instance, in the phrase "One, , buckle my shoe; three, four, open the door," the quantity is set up to the phrase "shoe," and the wide range 4 is attached to the phrase "door." This allows to create a mental picture that may be effects recalled.

2. Loci: Loci, or the "method of loci," is a mnemonic device that includes linking particular places to memories. For instance, if you want to remember a speech, you may link every issue to a specific place within the room. Then, whilst you supply the speech, you can look at every place to do not forget what you want to mention.

3. Story links: Story links incorporate telling your self a tale that connects the facts you need to keep in mind. As the tale progresses, the records becomes extra critical and much less tough to take into account.

four. Link: Linking consists of institutions among photos and the records you want to consider. For instance, you may hyperlink the photo of a light in your coffee maker to the engine mild on your vehicle to help you do not forget to make an appointment for vehicle safety within the morning.

These mnemonic techniques have precise techniques, but they percent a common purpose: growing sturdy institutions that might aid memory maintain in thoughts. These strategies can enhance your memory and help you don't forget statistics more with out troubles.

In addition to mnemonic strategies, there are other tactics to improve memory and increase mind flexibility. Here are some pointers:

1. Exercise: Regular workout has been showed to decorate mind characteristic and memory, and exercise will increase blood waft to the thoughts, that would enhance cognitive function.

2. Sleep: Getting sufficient sleep is crucial for reminiscence consolidation. During sleep, the thoughts consolidates recollections and strengthens neural connections.

3. Diet: A wholesome diet plan can enhance mind characteristic and reminiscence. Eating a diet wealthy in quit result, greens, and omega-3 fatty acids can assist decorate thoughts feature.

4. Mental stimulation: Engaging in mentally stimulating sports, which include puzzles, studying, and studying new abilties, can beautify thoughts function and memory.

Stress bargain: Chronic strain can harm mind function and reminiscence. Finding strategies to lessen strain, together with meditation, exercise, or spending time in nature, can enhance mind feature and reminiscence.

1. Practice: Like any potential, memory requires workout to decorate. Make a aware try to remember records, and use mnemonic techniques to resource recall.

2. Multitasking: Avoid multitasking as it could interfere with memory consolidation. Focus on one project at a time to beautify reminiscence remember.

three. Visualization: Visualizing statistics can make it less difficult to don't forget. Try to create shiny intellectual snap shots that may be with out trouble recalled.

four. Repetition: Repeating information can useful resource memory endure in mind. Repeat data numerous times, or use a spaced repetition approach, in which you evaluation facts at growing periods.

5. Emotion: Emotions may additionally moreover have a strong effect on reminiscence. Information that is related to robust emotions is much more likely to be remembered.

Memory is a dynamic manner that consists of the advent of latest neural connections. Improving memory consists of growing robust institutions that aid maintain in thoughts.

Mnemonic strategies, along side pegs, loci, tale hyperlinks, and linking, can efficaciously beautify memory take into account. In addition, ordinary workout, sufficient sleep, a healthful weight loss plan, intellectual stimulation, pressure bargain, exercise, visualization, repetition, and emotion can all useful resource memory preserve in mind. Incorporating the ones techniques into your every day existence can enhance your memory and enhance your mind flexibility.

Ways to Improve Memory

Many matters will can help you remember matters better. But you can not clearly do one detail to get the memory competencies you need and want. So, proper here are 9 easy techniques to help you recollect topics.

Consume a Balanced Diet

Just as you'll now not assume your automobile to artwork with out gas in the tank, you ought to not anticipate your mind to art work without gas. You want your thoughts to paintings similarly to it can.

Eating three well-balanced meals each day gives your thoughts the gasoline and building blocks to artwork at its pleasant. It's the splendid factor you may do to assist your brain bear in mind subjects.

A balanced meal has a protein, a complicated carbohydrate, and a fruit or a vegetable. Eating 3 properly-balanced food each day gives your mind the amino acids it wishes to make neurotransmitters, which is probably the chemical building blocks of your mind.

Each neurotransmitter allows you suspect and enjoy in strategies that make you satisfied and will let you undergo in thoughts. For instance, the neurotransmitter acetylcholine can be very important in your brain to take into account matters.

Get Enough Sleep

You need to preserve your thoughts calm and aware to apply your reminiscence talents absolutely. Getting sufficient sleep is the first-class way to get your self geared up to bear in mind.

If you do now not sleep enough, you may not be capable of pay interest prolonged sufficient to place what you want to preserve in thoughts into your thoughts. Attention is the vital issue to remembering matters. If you cannot pay interest, you may now not be able to open the gate. So preserve the gate open, loosen up, and get enough sleep.

Exercise Your Memory

Your frame has changed over many plenty and loads of years. To keep your body taking walks well, you need to workout session often. Your ancestors from lengthy inside the beyond did now not spend all day sitting in chairs or on couches.

Working out lets in your body and brain to preserve your organ systems strolling at their splendid. Working out quickens your coronary heart, metabolism, and meals glide in your mind. Exercise also makes it simpler to fall asleep at night time time time and lessens the stress you feel throughout the day. It will help you maintain your mind smooth and remember what you spot and pay interest.

Take Supplements (but Keep It Simple)

The biochemistry in your mind dreams nutrients, minerals, and herbal dietary supplements to work properly.

But dietary nutritional dietary supplements ought to by no means be considered an alternative to a healthful, well-balanced diet. Make certain to consume 3 nicely-balanced food each day. Think of nutritional dietary dietary supplements for what they will be: dietary supplements.

We stay in a society this is very focused on capsules, so do not believe that you want to take each complement that has been stated to decorate memory. But, then again, if you take too many nutritional dietary supplements and blend them with the drug treatments you're taking to deal with one in every of a kind ailments, you could have problems, like forgetting topics. So examine the rule of thumb "an lousy lot much less is more" in case you take dietary supplements.

Stick to the basics:

• Vitamin C

• Vitamin E

• Calcium and magnesium

• Omega-three fatty acid

• Multivitamin with all of the important Bs

Stimulate Your Mind

If you want to recall topics better, use your thoughts. Conversely, a lazy thoughts produces lazy reminiscence abilities.

You want to typically try and push yourself regardless of how antique you are. Through dendritic branching, your mind responds via making greater connections amongst your neurons. You'll additionally live alert and inquisitive about what goes on spherical you.

If you study too much TV, your brain will close to down. (Even reading academic indicates remains a passive manner to apply your mind.) Likewise, spend too much time considering what went incorrect in the course of the day, and you could not best make your self and those round you unhappy but moreover harm your memory because of the truth you may be preoccupied with subjects that don't be counted quantity.

Think of intellectual exercise as a manner to preserve your reminiscence skills in proper form. Get worried with the following:

• Read nonfiction books.

• Take education.

• Travel.

• Talk and argue about exciting things.

Develop Your Attention Span

Your memory wishes you to pay attention. Pay close to interest to do not forget. If you do no longer pay hobby, you may not be capable of positioned short-time period reminiscences into your prolonged-time period reminiscence. Do a few trouble you could to enhance your potential to pay interest. Focus on one issue for longer and longer quantities of time. Don't do many stuff without delay or transfer amongst them short. Let your self wander away in some aspect you need to do, and supply it your entire, undivided hobby. Set up a number of your regular activities so you'll be aware about every step you take to finish a assignment. Even if this makes you slower, think of it as an splendid exercise. You will not first-class work to decorate your capability to pay interest, but you could moreover find out that you cease your duties greater very well.

Stay Organized

If you preserve your self prepared, you'll be capable of don't forget what you want to take into account higher. Being organized does no longer suggest you want to be stiff; it approach having the capacity to inform your critiques aside and positioned them into classes that make feel.

If your lifestyles is a huge wide range, so will your memory. If you aren't prepared, you won't realise the way to discover your reminiscences; even worse, you may not have any memories to discover. So get matters in order so that you take into account to consider.

www.ingramcontent.com/pod-product-compliance
Lightning Source LLC
Chambersburg PA
CBHW051727020426
42333CB00014B/1189